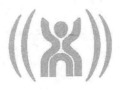

A Family's Guide To
TOURETTE SYNDROME

Editors:
Dr. J.T. Walkup, Dr. J.W. Mink, and
Dr. K. St. P. McNaught

CARNEGIE PUBLIC LIBRARY
202 N Animas St
Trinidad, CO 81082-2643
(719) 846-6841

iUniverse, Inc.
Bloomington

© Tourette Syndrome Association, Inc.

D0958656

A Family's Guide to Tourette Syndrome

Copyright © 2012 by Tourette Syndrome Association, Inc.

All rights reserved. No part of this book may be used or reproduced by any means, graphic, electronic, or mechanical, including photocopying, recording, taping or by any information storage retrieval system without the written permission of the publisher except in the case of brief quotations embodied in critical articles and reviews.

The information, ideas, and suggestions in this book are not intended as a substitute for professional medical advice. Before following any suggestions contained in this book, you should consult your personal physician. Neither the author nor the publisher shall be liable or responsible for any loss or damage allegedly arising as a consequence of your use or application of any information or suggestions in this book.

A Family's Guide to Tourette Syndrome may be ordered through iUniverse booksellers or by contacting:

iUniverse
1663 Liberty Drive   - or -
Bloomington, IN 47403
www.iuniverse.com
1-800-Authors (1-800-288-4677)

Tourette Syndrome Association, Inc.
42-40 Bell Blvd., Suite 205
Bayside, NY 11361
www.tsa-usa.org
718-224-2999

Because of the dynamic nature of the Internet, any web addresses or links contained in this book may have changed since publication and may no longer be valid. The views expressed in this work are solely those of the author and do not necessarily reflect the views of the publisher, and the publisher hereby disclaims any responsibility for them.

Any people depicted in stock imagery provided by Thinkstock are models, and such images are being used for illustrative purposes only.
Certain stock imagery © Thinkstock.

ISBN: 978-1-4620-6857-9 (sc)
ISBN: 978-1-4620-6858-6 (hc)
ISBN: 978-1-4620-6859-3 (ebk)

Library of Congress Control Number: 2012901967

Printed in the United States of America

iUniverse rev. date: 08/13/2012

CONTENTS

PREFACE

The national Tourette Syndrome Association, Inc. (TSA) was established in 1972 in Bayside, NY, by a group of parents seeking for themselves and for others a better understanding of what was then an obscure neurological disorder that was affecting their children. The organization has since grown dramatically and remains the only national, non-profit, membership organization of its kind in the U.S., and is now highly regarded internationally. Today, the TSA is arguably the most notable advocate for people touched by this disorder and is perhaps the leading supporter of Tourette syndrome research and education around the world.

During the phenomenal growth of the organization over the past 40 years, we remain committed to our original mission of seeking to increase and disseminate knowledge of Tourette syndrome among people who have the disorder, families, the general public, care providers, scientists, etc. Indeed, these individuals who we sought to serve, as well as many governmental and non-governmental organizations, have partnered in various ways with the TSA to advance the field of Tourette syndrome research and awareness. We also recognize the immeasurable contributions of our membership, generosity of our donors, commitment of our Board of Directors, and the hard work of the many scientists and clinicians, all of whom have a desire to see this complex disorder unraveled.

The TSA has traditionally provided medical and scientific information on the disorder in the form of brochures, newsletters, reprints of journal papers, articles written for us by experts in the field, and more. We will continue producing these sources of information along with this book which was conceived out of a need to consolidate these various publications into a single volume, written in non-technical/lay language, and is intended to become an authoritative and up-to-date source of information on Tourette syndrome for patients, families, schools, support groups, and the public at large.

The book is written by highly accomplished and leading neurologists, psychiatrists, psychologists, scientists and others with expertise in many areas of Tourette syndrome investigation and treatment. These individuals themselves have made significant contributions to our understanding of the disorder through research funded by the TSA and other organizations, as well as the NIH and the CDC. There is also a chapter in the book that is written by a mother who shares her experiences in helping her children cope with a disorder that is often difficult to treat with existing medications.

The TSA probably receives more requests for referrals and answers to medical/scientific questions on the disorder through our Information & Referrals service than for any other concern. Over the years, we have asked members of our Medical and Scientific Advisory Boards to respond to these questions in our official quarterly newsletter called *Inside TSA*. We have concluded this book with a selection of the top 50 frequently asked questions with answers which will be particularly helpful to individuals newly diagnosed with the disorder.

This book is the culmination of many years of commitment, support and research by many individuals touched by or interested in Tourette syndrome. We thank Dr. Arnold Lupin and the Lupin Foundation for their generosity in providing the funds to make this book possible. We hope that you find the information presented edifying, but recognize that this remains a work in progress and there is still much more that we need to learn about this complex disorder.

Reid Ashinoff, Chair, TSA Board of Directors

Judit Ungar, M.S.W., TSA President

FOREWORD

Dear Reader,

Well done! You made a great decision when you picked up a copy of this book, *A Family's Guide to Tourette Syndrome*. Before you plunge in and start turning pages, let me take a few moments of your time to tell you what you are in for. You have in your hands a unique resource for anyone concerned with Tourette syndrome. Perhaps you have thought that before—only to find either much less or much more than you wanted to read. But this time it is true, for this is neither another thumbnail of important topics nor a tome suitable only for doctors and researchers. This is something altogether new, an entirely readable but nonetheless comprehensive volume on all things Tourette, written for the well-informed layman.

Why target this group? Well, my life as a Tourette patient, neuroscientist, and long-time member of the Tourette Syndrome Association's Scientific Advisory Board has taught me that Tourette families are nothing if not well-informed! Quite often, the work of the TSA has helped to develop this body of educated laymen, the folks ready and able to learn more about the disorder and to take an active role in treatment, advocacy, and support of research. For decades now, a major part of TSA's mission has been to arm everyone they could reach with the facts about Tourette, and about living with it successfully. And here they are again, lashing together for this volume, a distinguished group of authors that includes many of the finest clinicians and researchers involved with Tourette. So, in 18 concise, authoritative chapters—here's what you have in store:

First, ten chapters cover everything you might want to know about Tourette in the clinical setting. These include a general introduction to Tourette, expert description of how the disorder is currently diagnosed, and what the best practices are for treatment with medication, cognitive behavioral therapy, and other modalities. Also covered are how Tourette treatment can be managed during pregnancy, and even how common we believe it to be, and how we have come to know that. On the research front, three chapters treat the latest results in the science of Tourette. These include a chapter on what makes the structure and function of the Tourette brain unique, another laying out our current knowledge of what the underlying genetic bases of the disorder might be, and the third describing what we understand about the role of autoimmune processes in development and exacerbation of Tourette.

But this volume transports us beyond the clinic and laboratory. Three chapters place Tourette in the context of the real world we live in. Two chapters review a wide range of psychosocial issues that Tourette patients encounter as they navigate the school and workplace environments throughout their lives. The third treats parenting a child with Tourette, from the perspective of a mother who has walked the walk.

The volume closes with a chapter containing dozens of frequently asked questions about Tourette, with concise answers written by experts, including many present or past members of the Tourette Syndrome Association's Scientific and Medical Advisory Boards.

As a neuroscientist whose Tourette symptoms appeared in the dark ages of the 1960s, I reviewed this volume with a sense of wonder! We cannot yet cure Tourette, but patients and their families—along with their friends, schoolmates and teachers—can navigate life successfully if we are armed with enough knowledge and insight. So start turning pages, you will find this book very useful.

Peter J. Hollenbeck, Ph.D.

CONTRIBUTORS

Editors

John T. Walkup, M.D.
Director, Division of Child & Adolescent
Psychiatry
Vice Chair, Department of Psychiatry
Weill Cornell Medical College & New York
Presbyterian Hospital
New York, NY

Jonathan W. Mink, M.D., Ph.D.
Professor of Neurology, Neurobiology,
& Anatomy and Pediatrics
Chief of Child Neurology
University of Rochester Medical Center
Rochester, NY

Kevin St. P. McNaught, Ph.D.
Vice President, Medical & Scientific Programs
Tourette Syndrome Association, Inc.
Bayside, NY

Managing Editor

Denise Walker, B.S.
Admin. Assistant, Medical & Scientific
Programs
Tourette Syndrome Association, Inc.
Bayside, NY

Editorial Assistants

Heather Cowley, Ph.D.
Manager, Medical & Scientific Programs
Tourette Syndrome Association, Inc.
Bayside, NY

Mariela Gutierrez, B.A.
Information & Referral Coordinator
Tourette Syndrome Association, Inc.
Bayside, NY

Agnes Njoh, M.S.
Project Coordinator
Tourette Syndrome Association, Inc.
Bayside, NY

Authors

Cheston M. Berlin, Jr., M.D.
Professor of Pediatrics
Penn State, Hershey
The Milton S. Hershey Medical Center
Hershey, PA

Michael H. Bloch, M.D., M.S.
Assistant Professor in Child Study Center
Assistant Director, Yale OCD Clinic
Department of Psychiatry
Yale Child Study Center
New Haven, CT

Cathy L. Budman, M.D.
Associate Professor of Psychology
Director, Movement Disorder Center, Psychiatry
Departments of Psychiatry & Neurology
North Shore University Hospital
LIJ Health System
Manhasset, NY

CONTRIBUTORS

Matthew R. Capriotti, B.S.
University of Florida
Department of Psychology
Gainesville, FL

Barbara J. Coffey, M.D., M.S.
Associate Professor, Child & Adolescent
Psychiatry
Director, Tics & Tourette's Clinical & Research
Program
New York University Child Study Center
New York University School of Medicine
New York, NY

Christine Erdie-Lalena, M.D.
Associate Professor of Pediatrics, University of
Washington & Seattle Children's Hospital (WA)
Assistant Professor, Uniformed services
University of the Health Sciences
Program Director of Developmental &
Behavioral Pediatrics
Fellowship @ Madigan Army Medical Center (WA)
Lieutenant Colonel in the U.S. Air Force (USAF)
Fort Lewis, WA

Flint M. Espil, M.S.
University of Florida
Gainesville, FL

Kelly D. Foote, M.D.
Associate Professor
Co-Director, Movement Disorders Center
Department of Neurosurgery
University of Florida
Gainesville, FL

Donald L. Gilbert, M.D., M.S.
Associate Professor of Child Neurology
Children's Division of Neurology
Director of Tourette Syndrome & Movement
Disorders Clinics
Cincinnati Children's Hospital Medical Center
Cincinnati, OH

Candy Hill, Ph.D.
Assistant Director of Research
Department of Psychiatry
University of Florida College of Medicine
Gainesville, FL

Peter J. Hollenbeck, Ph.D.
Former Co-chair of the TSA SAB
Professor and Associate Head of Biological
Sciences
Department of Biological Sciences
Purdue University
West Lafayette, IN

Joseph Jankovic, M.D.
Professor of Neurology
Distinguished Chair in Movement Disorders
Director, Parkinson's Disease Center &
Movement Disorders Clinic
Department of Neurology
Baylor College of Medicine
Houston, TX

Robert A. King, M.D.
Professor, Psychiatry
Professor in Child Study Center
Medical Director, Tourette's/OCD Clinic
Yale Child Study Center
New Haven, CT

James Leckman, M.D.
Neison Harris Professor of Child Psychiatry
& Pediatrics
Yale Child Study Center
Yale University School of Medicine
New Haven, CT

Irene Malaty, M.D.
Assistant Professor of Neurology
Medical Director of National Parkinson
Foundation Center of Excellence
Director of Tourette Syndrome Clinic
Department of Neurology
University of Florida
Gainesville, FL

Carol A. Mathews, M.D.
Associate Professor in Residence
Program for Genetics & Epidemiology of
Neuropsychiatric Symptoms
Department of Psychiatry
University of California, San Francisco
San Francisco, CA

Emilie R. Muelly, Ph.D.
Penn State, Hershey
The Milton S. Hershey Medical Center
Hershey, PA

Tanya Murphy, M.D., M.S.
Professor and the Maurice A. and Thelma P.
Rothman Endowed Chair
Director, Rothman Center for Pediatric
Neuropsychiatry at the Children's Health Center
within All Children's Hospital
Departments of Pediatrics & Psychiatry
University of South Florida
All Children's Hospital
St. Petersburg, FL

Michael S. Okun, M.D.
Associate Professor of Neurology
National Med. Dir. of National Parkinson
Foundation
Co-Director, Movement Disorders Center
Departments of Neurology, Neurosurgery,
Psychiatry and History
University of Florida
Gainesville, FL

Sue Levi-Pearl, B.A., M.A.
Emeritus Vice President, Medical &
Scientific Programs
Tourette Syndrome Association, Inc.
Bayside, NY

Nikki Ricciuti, RN, CCRC, LMHC
Research Coordinator
University of Florida
Department of Psychiatry
Gainesville, FL

**Mary M. Robertson, MBChB, M.D., DSc
(Med), DPM, FRCP, FRCPCH, FRCPsych**
Emeritus Professor of Neuropsychiatry
University College London
Visiting Professor & Honorary Consultant
Neuropsychiatrist, St. Georges Medical School
and Hospital
London, England

Lawrence Scahill, MSN, Ph.D.
Professor of Nursing & Child Psychiatry
Director of the Research Unit on Pediatric
Psychopharmacology
Yale University School of Nursing
Yale Child Study Center
New Haven, CT

Jeremiah M. Scharf, M.D., Ph.D.
Director of the Neurology Tic Disorders Clinic
Department of Neurology
Massachusetts General Hospital
Boston, MA

Elaine F. Shimberg, B.S., Honorary Ph.D.
Award Winning Author
Former National TSA Board Member
Past Chairman, St. Joseph's Hospital, (Tampa, FL)
Member, American Medical Writers Association
Member, American Society of Journalist and
Authors
Awarded Honorary Doctor of Humane Letters
Degree, University of South Florida
Tampa, FL

Herbert E. Ward, M.D.
Associate Professor of Psychiatry
Department of Psychiatry
University of Florida College of Medicine
Gainesville, FL

CONTRIBUTORS

Joanna Witkin, B.S.
Research Coordinator
North Shore University Hospital
LIJ Health System
Manhasset, NY

Douglas W. Woods, Ph.D.
Professor of Psychology
Director of Clinical Training
Department of Psychology
University of Wisconsin-Milwaukee
Milwaukee, WI

Samuel H. Zinner, M.D.
Associate Professor of Pediatrics
Director of Residency Training
Developmental Pediatrics
Center on Human Development & Disability
Department of Pediatrics
University of Washington School of Medicine
Seattle, WA

Amanda Zwilling, B.A.
Research Assistant at Langone Medical Center
New York University Child Study Center
New York University School of Medicine
New York, NY

ABBREVIATIONS

ABCT, Association for Behavioral and Cognitive Therapies
ADHD, Attention Deficit Hyperactivity Disorder
CAM, Complementary and Alternative Medicine
CBIT, Comprehensive Behavioral Intervention for Tics
CBT, Cognitive-Behavioral Therapy
CD, Conduct Disorder
CDC, Centers for Disease Control and Prevention
CNTNAP2, Contactin Associated Protein-like 2
CT, Chronic Tics
DBS, Deep Brain Stimulation
DNA, Deoxyribonucleic Acid
DSH, Deliberate Self-harm
DSM-IV, Diagnostic and Statistical Manual of Mental Disorders, Fourth Edition
DTI, Diffusion Tensor Imaging
FDA, Food and Drug Administration
GAS, Group A Streptococcus
ICD-10, International Classification of Diseases, Tenth Edition
IED, Intermittent Explosive Disorder
IEP, Individualized Education Program
IVIG, Intravenous Immunoglobulin
LD, Learning Disabled
MRI, Magnetic Resonance Imaging
NOSI, Non-Obscene Socially Inappropriate Behavior
OCB, Obsessive Compulsive Behaviors
OCD, Obsessive Compulsive Disorder
PANDAS, Pediatric Autoimmune Neuropsychiatric Disorders Associated with Streptococcus
QOL, Quality of Life
SIB, Self-injurious Behaviors
SLITRK1, SLIT and NTRK-like family, member 1
SSRIs, Selective Serotonin Reuptake Inhibitors
TD, Tourette Disorder
TS, Tourette Syndrome
TSA, Tourette Syndrome Association, Inc.
WHO, World Health Organization

CHAPTER 1

INTRODUCTION

Joseph Jankovic, M.D.

INTRODUCTION

In this introductory chapter, I try to provide a brief overview of TS with a focus on the most important topics. The subsequent chapters in this book, written by Tourette syndrome experts in an easy-to-understand language, will expand on the topics introduced here.

In 1885, Georges Albert Édouard Brutus Gilles de la Tourette, a 28 year old student of Jean-Martin Charcot, professor at the famous Salpêtrière Hospital in Paris and considered by many as the father of modern neurology, published "A Study of a Neurological Condition Characterized by Motor Incoordination Accompanied by Echolalia and Coprolalia". Gilles de la Tourette (abbreviated in the literature and in this book as Tourette) described 9 patients and noted that all shared one feature—they all exhibited brief involuntary movements, which we now call "motor tics". Additionally, 6 made noises, so called "vocal or phonic tics", 5 shouted obscenities, so called "coprolalia", 5 repeated the words of others, so called "echolalia", and 2 mimicked others' gestures, so called "echopraxia". Despite the recognition by his mentor, Charcot, and his professional accomplishments, Tourette lived a troubled personal life. Shortly after the tragic death of his young son, Tourette was shot in the head by a paranoid young woman. During the turn of the century, Tourette's behavior became erratic and bizarre, likely due to neurosyphilis, and his wife had to commit him to an asylum in Switzerland where he remained until his death in 1904.

Although Tourette considered the disorder he described to be hereditary, the cause was wrongly attributed to psychological causes for nearly a century following the original report. The perception of TS began to change in the 1960s when the beneficial effects of antipsychotic drugs, such as haloperidol, began to be recognized. This observation helped to change the view of the disorder from primarily "mental" to an organic, biological, disorder due to an abnormality of the brain circuitry involved in mediating motor and behavioral functions.

TICS

Tics, the clinical hallmark of TS, are relatively brief and intermittent movements (motor tics) or sounds (vocal or phonic tics). Currently accepted criteria for the diagnosis of TS require both types of tics, motor and phonic, to be present. This division into motor and phonic tics, however, is artificial, because the wide variety of sounds that TS patients make are actually motor tics that involve muscles of the nose, mouth, throat, and other structures besides the voice box (larynx). Therefore, the term "phonic" is preferable to the term "vocal" tic. Tics may be simple or complex. Simple motor tics involve only a small group of muscles, causing a movement that can be jerk-like ("clonic tic"), more sustained ("dystonic tic"), and in some cases the tic may be manifested by a simple contraction of a muscle ("tonic tic") or a brief cessation of motor activity ("blocking tic") without any accompanying movement. Examples of simple motor tics include blinking, nose twitching, mouth opening, head jerking, shoulder rotation, or tensing of abdominal or limb muscles. Complex motor tics consist of coordinated, sequenced movements resembling normal motor acts or gestures, such as touching, throwing, hitting, jumping, and kicking. Other examples of complex motor tics include inappropriate or obscene gesturing (copropraxia) or imitating other people's gestures (echopraxia). Burping, vomiting, retching, and air swallowing are also common forms of complex tics seen in patients with TS.

In addition to motor tics, patients with TS exhibit simple phonic tics, such as sniffing, throat clearing, grunting, squeaking, screaming, coughing, blowing, and sucking sounds. Patients may also have complex phonic tics such as coprolalia, echolalia, and repetition of one's own utterances, particularly the last syllable, word or phrase in a sentence, so called palilalia. Although many people mistakenly equate

TS with shouting of obscenities, coprolalia or copropraxia is present in only about 20% of all patients with TS.

One characteristic of a tic, which helps to differentiate this movement disorder from other abnormal involuntary movements, is the frequent presence of premonitory sensations, which precede tics in over 80% of TS patients. This premonitory phenomenon consists of sensations or discomforts, such as a burning feeling in the eye before an eye blink, tension or a crick in the neck that is relieved by stretching of the neck or jerking of the head, or a feeling of tightness or constriction that is relieved by extending an arm or leg. Many patients with TS are able to suppress their tics, for example while in public or in school or when playing video games, and release them when they are in a more comfortable environment, such as when not being observed or after returning home from school.

OTHER PROBLEMS ASSOCIATED WITH TS
In addition to tics, many patients with TS exhibit a variety of behavioral symptoms such as attention deficit with or without hyperactivity (ADHD), obsessive compulsive behavior or disorder (OCD), poor impulse control and many other behavioral problems, including oppositional defiant disorder, anxiety, depression, temper outbursts, rage attacks, self-injuries, and inappropriate sexual behavior. These and other behavioral comorbidities are discusses in subsequent chapters in this book.

MISCONCEPTIONS
There are many misconceptions about TS, not only stemming from its misclassification as a "mental" disorder. For example, traditional descriptions of tics often stated that the movements and noises disappear during sleep. This is not the case as researchers have demonstrated by all-night sleep and brain wave electroencephalogram recordings (polysomnography) that tics may persist during all stages of sleep. Another misconception is that TS occurs only in children. While the diagnostic definition, currently still based on the Diagnostic and Statistical Manual of Mental Disorders, Fourth Edition, which is currently under revision and DSM-5 is expected to be released soon, requires that tics start before the age of 18 years, TS can clearly

persist into or recur in adulthood. In fact, most tics in adults represent recurrences of childhood tics.

CAN TICS BE HARMFUL?

Tics, although rarely disabling, can be quite troublesome for TS patients because they cause embarrassment, interfere with social interactions, and at times can be quite painful or uncomfortable. Rarely, neck tics may be so forceful and violent, the so-called "whiplash tics", that they may cause neurologic deficits, such as carotid artery dissection, and secondary spine changes associated with compression of the spinal cord. Patients, parents and physicians must be aware of these potentially dangerous tics as these represent neurologic emergencies and must be treated promptly.

THE PROGNOSIS

The natural history of TS is quite variable, but on the average, tics (and ADHD) usually first appear around the age of 6 years and usually become most severe at age 10, just before puberty. All symptoms usually spontaneously improve by 18 years of age at which time about half of the patients become tic-free. Although tics and ADHD usually markedly improve by late teens, OCD symptoms tend to persist into adulthood and in some cases tics re-emerge in middle or older age.

FREQUENCY

Although the worldwide prevalence of TS has been reported to range from 0.3% to 0.8% of all children, some epidemiological studies suggest that up to 24% of children may have tics sometime during their childhood, and up to 2-3% of all children develop some features of TS.

CAUSE(S)

TS is one of the most common genetic disorders of childhood, but the causative gene or genes have not yet been identified. Mutations in two genes, the Slit and NTRK-like family, member 1 gene on chromosome 13 and the L-histidine decarboxylase gene on chromosome 15, recently have been reported to cause TS, but when studied in large populations of TS patients, no abnormalities have been found in these genes, suggesting that they account for a very small proportion of all patients with TS.

Besides genetic causes, there are many other reasons why some people develop tics and other symptoms of TS, sometimes referred to as "tourettism". These include infection, head trauma, stroke, multiple sclerosis, cocaine and other drugs, cerebral palsy, autistic disorders, and many other causes.

The exact mechanism of tics and the various behavioral comorbidities is not known but the weight of evidence from a large body of laboratory and clinical research supports the hypothesis that TS arises from abnormalities in the brain circuitry that primarily involves the surface of the brain, called cortex, and deep brain structures called the basal ganglia. It has been hypothesized that as a result of genetic and other abnormalities the connections between these brain areas are disrupted, leading to loss of inhibition or disinhibition of normal motor and behavioral brain pathways.

ABNORMALITIES IN THE BRAINS OF PATIENTS

Only a few brains of patients with TS have been studied at autopsy. Detailed examination of these brains found essentially no abnormalities except for some evidence of mild cell loss, but this requires further study and confirmation. Biochemical studies have shown some subtle abnormalities in certain neurotransmitters and receptors, but no consistent changes have been identified.

ARE THERE ANY TESTS THAT CAN BE DONE TO DIAGNOSE TS?

The diagnosis of TS is based strictly on clinical criteria and there is no laboratory test that indicates or confirms the diagnosis. Blood tests are rarely needed to exclude other causes of tics, such as prior streptococcal infection or red blood cell abnormality called acanthocytosis. Likewise, brain wave electroencephalogram or brain scan Magnetic Resonance Imaging is almost never needed in the evaluation of patients suspected of TS unless there are some neurological abnormalities identified on examination. Although standard MRIs are usually normal, some studies evaluating large groups of patients with TS have identified some subtle changes. For example, instead of the left side of the brain being larger than the right side, the two sides are the same size.

TREATMENTS

The treatment of TS must be individualized and tailored to the specific needs of each patient and not every patient with TS requires therapy. The patient, parents, teachers, counselors, and physician must work as partners in selecting the best school or work environment for the patient in order to optimize productivity and achieve full potential. This might include extra break periods and a refuge area to allow the release of tics, waiving time limitations on tests or adjusting timing of tests to the morning, and other measures designed to relieve stress. National and local support groups can provide additional information and can serve as a valuable resource for the patient and his or her family (www. tsa-usa.org).

Before discussing treatments with medications, a few remarks about behavioral therapy. The Comprehensive Behavioral Intervention for Tics (CBIT) disorders, primarily based on utilization of habit reversal therapy, a technique that employs competing-response training teaches the patient to initiate a voluntary behavior to manage the premonitory urge, has been recently found effective in 2 controlled clinical trials. The success of this behavioral management is critically dependent on active involvement by the parents and the therapist, both of whom must be well trained and skilled in the various CBIT techniques.

While behavioral therapy may be helpful for some patients, those whose symptoms are troublesome and interfere with daily functioning or social interaction may require medications to manage their symptoms. All medications should be instituted at low doses and gradually increased in an attempt to find the optimal dosage. Another important principle of therapy in TS is to give each medication an adequate time before the dosage is adjusted or before it is concluded that the drug is not effective. Although selection of appropriate drug should be based on evidence derived from placebo-controlled studies, such clinical trials are often lacking and, therefore, personal experience of the physician often drives the selection of the drug. The following drugs have been found to be useful in the treatment of tics: fluphenazine, risperdal, and tetrabenazine. Although not yet studied in large clinical trials or approved by the Food and Drug Administration, tetrabenazine is gradually emerging as an effective and safe drug in the treatment of tics. The drug is well tolerated, but some patients experience drowsiness, depression, insomnia, and restlessness. Its main advantage over the conventional anti-tic medications, such as haloperidol and pimozide, the only two drugs currently approved by the Food and Drug Administration for the treatment of TS, is that it does not cause tardive dyskinesia. Other drugs used in the treatment of tics include clonidine, guanfacine, clonazepam and topiramate. Motor tics, particularly if they are localized to only one area (such as blinking, facial grimacing, neck tics) may be successfully treated with botulinum toxin injections in the affected muscles.

Central nervous system stimulants, such as methylphenidate, dexmethylphenidate, methamphetamine, dextroamphetamine, levoamphetamine, pemoline, and lisdexamfetamine dimesylate are clearly the most effective agents in the treatment of ADHD. Although imipramine and desipramine have been reported to be useful in the treatment of OCD, the most effective drugs are the selective serotonin reuptake inhibitors, such as fluoxetine, fluvoxamine, clomipramine, paroxetine, sertraline, venlafaxine, citalopram, and escitalopram. Surgical treatment of TS using deep brain stimulation should be reserved only for patients with disabling symptoms unresponsive to medical therapy.

CHAPTER 2

THE DIAGNOSIS OF TOURETTE SYNDROME

James F. Leckman, M.D., Michael H. Bloch, M.D.,
and Robert A. King, M.D.

INTRODUCTION

In this chapter, we discuss the key clinical features of TS. This is important for several reasons. First, our understanding of this condition and related disorders has increased a great deal over the past 30 to 40 years, and it is important to become familiar with what is known about key aspects of the symptoms of TS. Second, if you are looking at this book, you are probably wondering if someone you know has TS. This chapter will describe what TS looks like from the outside and how it feels on the inside. We will also cover how the condition typically changes over an individual's lifetime.

WHAT ARE TICS?

Tics are often more easily recognized than precisely defined. Tics are sudden, rapid, motor movements or sounds that recur. Usually, tics can be easily mimicked and they can be confused with normal movements or sounds. They have a "stereotyped" quality which simply means that the tic looks or sounds more or less the same each time it occurs. Tics can be thought of as fragments of normal behavior that appear without any logical reason. Tics can be easily mimicked and they can be confused with normal movements or sounds. If the observer (a parent, teacher, or a peer) does not know better, they may think that tics are being done "on purpose." This can be very problematic as we discuss below.

Tics are described based on their anatomical location, number, frequency, and duration. Another useful descriptor is the intensity or "forcefulness" of the tic, as some tics call attention to themselves simply by virtue of their exaggerated, forceful character. Finally, tics are also described in terms of their "complexity." "Simple tics" are sudden, brief (usually less than 1 second in duration), meaningless movements or sounds. "Complex tics" are sudden, more purposive appearing, stereotyped movements of longer duration that can include "orchestrated" combinations of motor or vocal, or motor and vocal, tics. The observed range of tics is extraordinary, so that virtually any voluntary motor movement or vocalization can emerge as a tic. Table 1 presents a brief compendium of some of the more common motor and vocal tics sorted by how "complex" the tics are.

Table 1: Examples of simple and complex motor and vocal tics

Tic Symptoms	Examples
Simple Motor Tics: *Sudden, brief, meaningless movements*	Eye blinking, eye movements, grimacing, nose twitching, mouth movements, lip pouting, head jerks, shoulder shrugs, arm jerks, abdominal tensing, kicks, finger movements, jaw snaps, tooth clicking, rapid jerking of any part of the body
Complex Motor Tics: *Slower, longer, more "purposeful" movements*	Sustained "looks," facial gestures, biting, touching objects or self, throwing, banging, thrusting arms, gestures with hands, gyrating and bending, dystonic postures (holding an uncomfortable pose), copropraxia (obscene gestures)

Simple Phonic Tics: *Sudden, meaningless, sounds or noises*	Throat clearing, coughing, sniffling, spitting, screeching, barking, grunting, gurgling, clacking, hissing, sucking, and innumerable other sounds
Complex Phonic Tics: *Sudden, more "meaningful" utterances*	Syllables, words, phrases, statements such as "shut up," "stop that," "oh, okay," "I've got to," "okay honey," "what makes me do this?," "how about it," or "now you've seen it," speech atypicalities (usually rhythms, tone, accents, intensity of speech); echo phenomenon (immediate repetition of one's own or another's words or phrases); and coprolalia (obscene, inappropriate, and aggressive words and statements)

Complex tics are rarely observed in the absence of simple tics. Within the larger group of complex tics there are specific forms of tics that have their own names. Some complex motor movements are considered **dystonic tics,** which are a set of sustained muscle contractions that can cause twisting movement of the body, resulting in an abnormal posture. Gilles de la Tourette in his original description was intrigued by a range of complex tics including the imitation of gestures (**echopraxia**) or sounds or words (**echolalia**). Doctors call the rude or obscene gestures with hands or tongue "**copropraxia**" and the uttering of obscenities or rude speech "**coprolalia**". Self-injurious complex tics (hitting the face, biting a hand or wrist) are rarely observed in those with TS. Unfortunately, these tics are often featured in the media (talk shows, movies, etc.) because of their sensational character and leave the unsuspecting public with an incorrect impression of what TS is.

PREMONITORY SENSORY URGES AND THAT "FLEETING AND INCOMPLETE SENSE OF RELIEF"

Tics are temporarily suppressible and often preceded by a **premonitory urge** which is similar to the sensation prior to a sneeze or the itch that leads to a scratch. Individuals describe premonitory urge as the buildup of tension in a particular body location. Examples of premonitory urges include the feeling of having something in one's throat, or a localized discomfort in the shoulders, leading to the need to clear one's throat or shrug the shoulders, respectively. Depending on the intensity of the urge, the individual may consciously decide to tic or not to tic. However, if the urge is very strong, it can be perceived as impossible to resist and may even become the reason a person with TS gives for ticcing. The actual tic may be felt as relieving this tension or sensation, similar to scratching an itch. After the tic is done, there is often a fleeting and incomplete sense of relief. It is also important to note that young children under the age of 10 years do not report these urges. It is unknown if the urges actually develop later in the course of the disorder, or young children are unaware of these urges like they are sometimes unaware of their tics.

The neck, shoulder girdle, throat, hands, the midline of the stomach, the front of the thighs and the feet are "hot spots" for premonitory urges (Figure 1). For some, the urges are located in a small discrete area that can be readily identified. For others, these urges are more generalized and are best described by a sense of inner tension. Many individuals will report having both types of sensations. These sensory urges have also been described as sensory tics. Just because an individual may have some premonitory urges does not mean that every tic is preceded by such an urge. Often tics involving more automatic behaviors, like eye blinking, do not have urges that precede them.

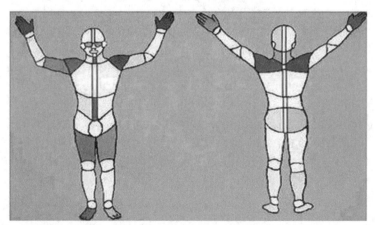

Figure 1. Density of Premonitory Urges. The densities of premonitory urges for 89 anatomical regions are depicted. The areas with highest density are darker in color. From: Leckman JF, Walker DE, Cohen DJ: Premonitory urges in Tourette syndrome, Am J Psychiatry 1993; 150:98-102.

The association of premonitory urges with the sense of relief after tic completion is a key element in one of the behavioral treatments that have been shown to be effective for TS. Originally called Habit Reversal Training and developed by Nathan Azrin in the 1970s, the behavioral treatment has been adapted and is currently called a Comprehensive Behavioral Intervention for Tics. The initial phase of Habit Reversal Training and Comprehensive Behavioral Intervention for Tics is "awareness training," where the individual learns to become more acutely aware of the type and nature of their tics, premonitory urges, and what environments or experiences make tics better and worse.

SENSATIONS WITHOUT SOURCES

Many individuals with TS are remarkably sensitive to experiences in their daily life which trigger ticcing and may give the impression that tics are voluntary. As first noted by Gilles de la Tourette and described above, individuals may mirror the behavior (echopraxia) and speech (echolalia) of others as well as of themselves (palilalia). People with TS may tic in response to something they have just seen or heard. This is especially problematic if a child at school echoes his teacher's admonition to "sit down" or "stop talking". Specific environmental events can also trigger tics. For example, tags in t-shirts or underwear, constricting clothing, such as turtle neck sweaters and tight collars, or elasticity in the ribs in socks can trigger tics and related movements. Other individuals report the emergence of urges to perform more complex acts that are dangerous, forbidden, or simply senseless and bizarre in response to proscriptive injunctions. It is not uncommon for a patient to feel like he or she has to touch the center of a hot frying pan on the stove, run a finger along a sharp knife, put the car in reverse gear while driving down a highway, touch someone or shout out in a quiet church service. Those individuals with stimulus-bound tics may also report the distress and frustration over the unwitting acts of others that may provoke their tic symptoms; for example, a person's cough or gesture may set off a bout of tics in response.

It is possible that symptoms we associate with the Obsessive Compulsive Disorder may belong in this category (see Chapter 3: Psychiatric Conditions Associated with TS). Some of the "just right" phenomena, e.g., the need for things to be arranged over and over again until they look just right and when a person describes ticcing a certain number of times or in a particular way to satisfy the internal urge may be related to this sensitivity to triggering experiences.

WHAT IS REALLY GOING ON WITH PREMONITORY URGES?

In our view, understanding these premonitory sensory urges is important. It is not only important for those who suffer with TS, but also for parents, teachers and friends. TS is more than just the movements and sounds. It is characterized clinically by a loss of the brain's "automatic" ability to suppress or "gate" irrelevant sensory information that arises in the body or in an individual's physical surroundings.

Understanding the sensory component of tics and TS can be enormously helpful to parents, as well as other family members, teachers and other children. The movements and sounds at times seem "strange" or "weird," but what if the person is doing it only because he or she feels something like the need to scratch or cough? In our experience, this gives everyone a chance to understand something of what it is like to have tics.

It will also be important for doctors and scientists to understand where these sensations are coming from as this may be a key element in understanding why TS exists in the first place. Peter J. Hollenbeck, Ph.D., a Professor of Biological Sciences who has TS (see **Foreword**) said it this way:

"I finally apprehend the magnitude of the background noise that I have been experiencing for decades . . . the people around me do not share my tics because they do not hear the drumbeat. They do not feel the sensations without sources; do not have irresistible urges to pause in mid-sentence . . . and so on in endless, bewildering variety . . . Finally and most important, I feel convinced that this complex challenging enigmatic internal world is the obvious core of Tourette."

THINGS THAT MAKE TICS BETTER OR WORSE

Table 2 provides a list of things that can make tics better or worse. This varies from person to person. There are a few things to remember when you look over this list. First, it is good to be prepared and to know ahead of time about situations where the tics may be more noticeable. However, as a general rule, for children it is better *not to avoid* situations that are part of normal development even if the tics would be more noticeable; for example, birthday parties or school performances. It is far better to keep a child's development on track than to try to avoid situations where the tics will be worse.

Second, for parents and teachers, one of the other lessons that it is important to learn is that if you tell a child to "Stop doing that!" you are simply setting the stage for more tics to come out as you are making the child more anxious and self-conscious. Similarly, if you are always asking about the tics or the premonitory urges, more tics will appear. Sometimes tics that have been gone for a long time can reappear.

Third, knowing when the tics will be bad will help many individuals figure out strategies to counter the tics. One of our patients would regularly ask her father to go play ping pong with her in the basement. Another would just plan to go play his flute. It is also possible that when someone gets really good at the behavioral treatments for tics that it is nothing more than "Doing something that requires focused attention and motor control" (Table 2).

Table 2: What makes tics better or worse?

Better	Sleep (almost always the tics will be reduced or disappear) Doing something that requires focused attention and motor control, like riding a bicycle or playing ping pong or playing a musical instrument (almost always) During and after physical exercise (usually the tics will diminish or be less forceful)
Worse	Excitement, like going off to Disney World for the first time, birthdays, holidays especially with presents (almost always) Being anxious or upset or noticing stress in a loved one (almost always) Watching exciting movies (in the theater) or television shows (almost always) Being tired, but not quite ready to fall asleep (almost always) Being alone (almost always) Being sick or being injured (almost always) Asking about or imitating a person's tics, tics are "suggestible" (almost always) Menstruation (only for some women) Eating (only for some individuals) Drinking coffee (only for some individuals) Being too hot, hot weather (only for some individuals)

IS IT POSSIBLE NOT TO TIC?

Yes, people can briefly suppress their tics, but the waxing and waning of tics in different environments/circumstances is more than just suppressing or "letting go." It is likely due to a number of factors, like the nature of the activity in which the person is involved and the person's mental state. The fact that tics come and go can be confusing to those who know or work with a child or adult with TS. For example, teachers sometimes think that because the child is not ticcing when engaged in a calm focused activity, but all of a sudden starts ticcing again when engaged in an exciting school activity, that the child is *in control* of his or her ticcing. So they conclude that when the child is not ticcing, he/she is consciously suppressing tics and when he/she starts ticcing, that he/she is "letting it go" or doing it to annoy or frustrate the teacher's efforts in the classroom. One of the common patterns of tics that bother parents is the observation that kids don't appear to tic much at school but when they get home the tics explode. The presumption is the child has suppressed his tics all day and then "lets them go" at home. It is also likely that fewer tics at school and more at home after school is a function of the child being engaged in calm mental activities at school and when they got home they were excited and enjoying the freedom of being out of school. Getting the word out about what makes tics better and worse is very important for those with TS, their families, teachers, peers, and coworkers. This knowledge often goes a long way in helping people with TS live successfully with others (see Chapter 15: Living with TS).

THE DIAGNOSIS

There is no sensitive and specific set of diagnostic tests for TS or other tic disorders at present. The diagnosis is based solely on the individual's history and clinical presentation. Consequently, the current diagnostic classifications of tic disorders are based on the conventional wisdom of experts in the field, their experience as clinicians, as well as the available scientific literature.

The most frequently used system for diagnosis in the United States is the American Psychiatric Association's Diagnostic and Statistical Manual of Mental Disorders. It now exists in its fourth edition and is often referred to as DSM-IV. The diagnoses in DSM-IV and the code numbers assigned to each of these diagnoses are used for a number of different purposes including research, record keeping, public health records, and insurance reimbursement. The DSM-IV also uses the same code numbers as the International Classification of Diseases (ICD) which is now in its tenth edition (ICD-10).

DSM-IV and ICD are currently in the midst of being revised by committees of researchers, scientists, and clinicians. These criteria, like the descriptions offered by Gilles de la Tourette, have focused on cataloguing and classifying tics as viewed from the outside. Although we don't anticipate big changes in the diagnostic criteria, we don't believe that everyone with a diagnosis of TS has the same underlying brain condition. Right now we are limited in our understanding of how the brain is involved in ticcing (see Chapters 6 and 7: The Cause(s) of TS and Changes that Occur in the Brain and Inheritance, Genes and TS, respectively). This is an important point. As human beings we think "categorically": Does my child have Tourette or not? I want to know and it really matters in terms of what happens in school and for my insurance company. So, does my child have TS or not? This is a simple question, but at the level of biology and the brain, it is not so simple; not everyone's TS is necessarily the same.

IMPAIRMENT

Impairment is partly dependent on frequency, intensity, complexity, and duration of specific tics. Estimates of impairment also need to include the impact on the individual's self-esteem, family life, social acceptance, school or job functioning, and physical well-being. For example, a very frequent simple motor wrist tic may be less impairing than an infrequently occurring, forceful copropraxic gesture. Also, some people cope better with their tics than others. What might be a mild tic for one person, might be difficult for another person. It is not uncommon early in the course of TS for the child and parents to fear what the future may be and unwittingly make a child more uncomfortable and the tics worse. Most of the time, as people become older, they and their families understand their symptoms better and cope more successfully. However, as people with TS age, they may be more acutely aware of their tics and their impact on other people, setting the stage for either anxiety, distress or both and a secondary worsening of tics. Coping is also dependent on other conditions the person with TS may have, such as ADHD, OCD or other anxiety or mood disorders; these conditions by their nature cause impairment and also undermine a person's ability to cope with their tics. Older individuals with TS are often acutely aware of their tics and their impact on other people, setting the stage for either anxiety and distress or a determined effort to be a "self-advocate." The stress and anxiety can lead to a vicious cycle that can have serious detrimental effects on self-esteem and limit socialization, which can in turn lead to more severe tics.

THE TIMING OF TICS

The DSM criteria mention "waxing and waning." This is a very important feature of tics. This simply means that over a period of weeks to months, a person's tics get better or worse. We still do not understand exactly why this happens. For children, tics increase at the start of school, during the winter holidays, or on vacation. TS may be due to seasonal patterns of excitement or stress and become predictable over time. But it may also be due to the brain circuits and the biology of the brain cells that regulate those circuits.

Individual tics tend to occur in "bouts." A bout is a brief, or not so brief, series of tics with relatively regular inter-tic intervals that can be measured in seconds or even fractions of a second. These bouts themselves occur in bouts and may account for transient periods of tic exacerbation that occur during the course of a typical day. Few scientific studies have focused on the timing of tics. But speculation has focused on the "fractal" occurrence of tics. This fractal quality means that regardless of the time increments studied, seconds, minutes, hours, days, weeks, or years, the nonlinear temporal patterning of tics or bouts of tics or bouts-of-bouts of tics or bouts-of-bouts-of-bouts of tics or bouts-of-bouts-of-bouts-of-bouts of tics remains basically the same (Figure 2). This quality, if confirmed, may elucidate a fundamental property of tics and tic disorders.

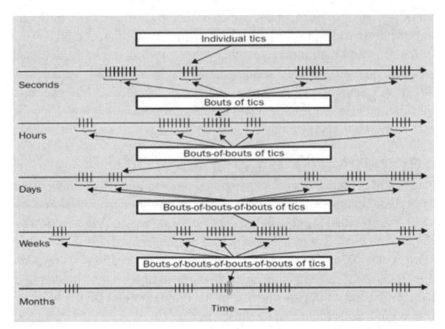

Figure 2. Leckman JF. Tourette syndrome. Lancet 2002; 360:1577-1586; Peterson BS, Leckman JF: Temporal characterization of tics in Gilles de la Tourette syndrome. Biol Psychiatry 1998; 44:1337-1348.

Tics then might be best understood as being the product of nested processes that unfold over many time scales, from milliseconds to years or even decades. This brings us to the next important topic, the natural course of Tourette.

Subsequently, the classic history includes a waxing and waning course and a changing repertoire of tics. Typically, in cases of TS, the symptoms multiply and worsen so that even during the waning phases the tics are troublesome. Importantly, for a majority of individuals, the period of worst ever tic severity usually falls between the ages of 7 and 15 years following which there is a steady decline in tic severity. The average age of a person's worst tic presence is usually close to 11 years (Figure 4). The fall off in tic symptoms is consistent with available epidemiological data that indicate a lower prevalence of TS among adults compared to children (see Chapter 5: How Common Is TS in Children). It is also typical of the findings in our follow-up studies of individuals that we first met as children and who we sought out in early adulthood to see how they were doing. In many instances, the vocal tics become increasingly rare or may disappear altogether.

In adulthood, a patient's repertoire of tics usually diminishes in size and becomes predictable during periods of fatigue and heightened emotionality. Complete remission of both motor and phonic symptoms has also been reported; estimates vary considerably with some studies reporting rates of remission as high as 50%. In such cases, the legacy of TS in adult life is most closely associated with what it "meant" to have severe tics as a child. For example, the individual who was misunderstood and punished at home and at school for their tics or who was teased mercilessly by peers will fare worse than a child whose interpersonal environment was more understanding and supportive and who coped well and who was encouraged to become a self-advocate and to not be ashamed of their tics.

In contrast, adulthood is also the period when the most severe and debilitating forms of tic disorder can be seen. In this small minority of adults severe tics can persist or evolve. At their worst, these tics can be self-injurious and disabling, substantially impacting adult functioning.

THE NATURAL HISTORY OF TICS AND TIC DISORDERS

Tics usually have their onset in the first decade of life. Most investigators report a median onset of simple motor tics at five or six years of age.

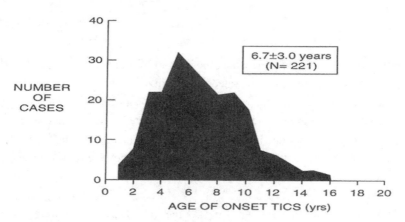

Figure 3. Age of Onset Distribution. From: Leckman JF, Cohen DJ: Tourette Syndrome: Tics, Obsessions, Compulsions—Developmental Psychopathology and Clinical Care. New York: John Wiley and Sons, 1998.

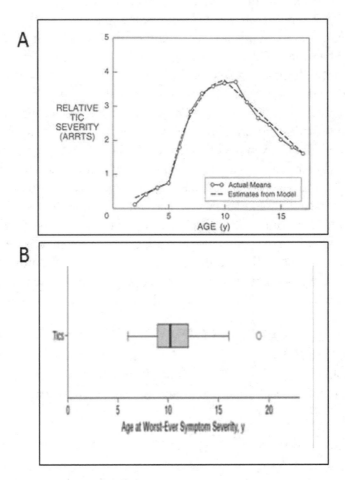

Figure 4. Course of Tic Severity over the First Two Decades

A. Relative severity of tics is presented for 42 individuals with Tourette syndrome (A-D). The relative tic severity scale goes from 0 (no tics) to 5 (severe tics). Estimates from the patient and a respective parent were obtained independently. From: Leckman JF, Zhang H, Vitale A, Lahnin F, Lynch K, Bondi C, Kim Y-S, Peterson BS. Course of tic severity in Tourette syndrome: The first two decades. Pediatrics 1998; 102:14-19.

B. Box plot representing age when tic disorder (OCD) symptoms were at their worst (N=46).
From: Bloch MH, Peterson BS, Scahill L, Otka J, Katsovich L, Zhang H, Leckman JF. Clinical predictors of future tic and OCD severity in children with Tourette syndrome Arch Pediatrics Adolesc Med, 2006; 160:65-69.

NOT EVERYONE'S TS OR "DISORDER" IS THE SAME

Global outcome and social and career capacities in adulthood are not synonymous with tic outcomes. The major reason for this discrepancy is that a majority of individuals with TS also suffer from related disorders. In addition to tics, many patients with TS have symptoms of attention-deficit hyperactivity disorder, obsessive-compulsive disorder, or both, and a range of other mood and anxiety disorders (see Chapter 3: Psychiatric Conditions Associated with TS). These coexisting disorders can add greatly to morbidity associated with TS and detract from the individual's overall quality of life. Increased irritability and rage attacks associated with anxiety and mood disorders are not so uncommon among patients with TS (Chapter 4: Problems with Anger, Aggression, and Impulse Control in TS). Strikingly, in population-based studies, these co-occurring disorders occur more commonly in individuals who met the full criteria for TS. Individuals with Chronic Motor or Vocal Tic Disorder are much less likely to be affected by these symptoms compared to those with TS. When additional disorders are present the individual's quality of life is usually poorer, and the level of overall impairment is usually much greater than if the individual just meets the criteria for TS.

WHAT TO LOOK FOR IN AN EVALUATION AND SOME PARTING THOUGHTS

The clinical evaluation of a person with TS properly considers the "whole person," possessed of a rich personal and interpersonal life, not just a collection of abnormal sensory urges and tic symptoms. In the process of a comprehensive evaluation, the full range of difficulties and competencies should be charted, beginning with the individual child's or adult's strengths and interests. Despite the availability of effective behavioral interventions and medication treatments (see Chapters 9 and 11: Drug Treatments Latest Treatments & Related Issues for TS and Behavioral Therapy, respectively), we consistently find substantial benefit from encouraging individuals and families to build on their child's strengths.

Apart from building on the individual's strengths and keeping their development and function on track, a critical question is the degree to which tics interfere with the child's emotional, social, familial, and school/work experiences. To determine this, it is often useful to monitor symptoms over a few months to assess their severity and the capacity of the person with TS, their family, peers, and coworkers to adapt and cope.

At the time of evaluation, the person with TS may be upset by his or her inability to control the tics and by criticism from parents, teachers, coworkers and peers who exhort him or her to control his or her strange behavior, which they may believe he or she can control. Although it is easy to focus on the upsetting and socially stigmatizing tics, it is the clinician's responsibility to place the tics into the proper context of the person's overall development and function. Indeed, the diagnostic evaluation, by providing important information and correcting misconception, establishes the building blocks of a successful treatment.

Acknowledgement: This chapter is dedicated to the memory of Donald J. Cohen who founded the Yale Tic Disorders Clinic more than 35 years ago and the many individuals and families whom we have evaluated and followed over this period of time. Add to this the many clinicians and researchers who have been trained in the clinic and subsequently gone on to become leaders in this field.

References

1. Bloch, M.H., Peterson, B.S., Scahill, L., Otka, J., Katsovich, L., Zhang, H. & Leckman, J.F. (2006) Clinical predictors of future tic and OCD severity in children with Tourette syndrome *Arch Pediatr Adolesc Med* **160**, 65-69.
2. Gorman, D.A., Thompson, N., Plessen, K.J., Robertson, M.M., Leckman, J.F. & Peterson, B.S. (2010) A controlled follow-up study of psychosocial outcome and psychiatric comorbidity in young adults with Tourette syndrome. *Br J Psychiatry* **197**, 36–44.
3. Leckman, J.F. (2002) Tourette syndrome. *Lancet* **360**, 1577-1586.
4. Leckman, J.F. & Cohen, D.J. (1998) *Tourette Syndrome: Tics, Obsessions, Compulsions – Developmental Psychopathology and Clinical Care.* John Wiley and Sons, NY.
5. Leckman, J.F., Riddle, M.A., Hardin, M.T., Ort, S.I., Swartz, K.L., Stevenson, J., & Cohen, D.J. (1989) The Yale Global Tic Severity Scale (YGTSS): Initial testing of a clinician rated scale of tic severity. *J Am Acad Child Adolesc Psychiatry* **28**, 566 573.
6. Leckman, J.F., Walker, D.E. & Cohen, D.J. (1993) Premonitory urges in Tourette syndrome. *Am J Psychiatry* **150**, 98-102.
7. Leckman, J.F., Zhang, H., Vitale, A., Lahnin, F., Lynch, K., Bondi, C., Kim, Y.S. & Peterson, B.S. (1998) Course of tic severity in Tourette syndrome: The first two decades. *Pediatrics* **102**, 14-19.
8. Peterson, B.S. & Leckman, J.F. (1998) Temporal characterization of tics in Gilles de la Tourette syndrome. *Biol Psychiatry* **44**, 1337-1348.

CHAPTER 3

PSYCHIATRIC CONDITIONS ASSOCIATED WITH TOURETTE SYNDROME

Barbara J. Coffey, M.D., M.S. and Amanda Zwilling, B.A.

INTRODUCTION

Psychiatric conditions co-occurring with TS, known as comorbid disorders, have long been described in association with the condition. Gilles de la Tourette himself reported that several of his patients had "fears, phobias and arithmomania," which would now be described as obsessive-compulsive symptoms. Historically, investigators have reported elevated rates of anxiety, phobias, panic attacks and generalized anxiety disorder in TS patients[1,62]. Today, however, the nature of the relationship between TS and the frequently observed psychiatric comorbid disorders in clinically referred individuals has yet to be definitively disentangled. Obsessive-compulsive symptoms, developmentally inappropriate motoric hyperactivity and inattention, worry and fears, depressed mood, irritability and aggressive dyscontrol have often been described in association with TS. Given the underlying central core disinhibition or dysregulation in the central nervous system pathways involved in TS, it is reasonable to assume that in addition to motor and vocal symptoms, behavioral and emotional dysfunction may be characteristic of some with the disorder.

Although estimates of the prevalence of co-occurring psychiatric disorders in TS patients vary from setting to setting, most studies report high prevalence rates, some as high as 90% in clinically referred samples[2-3]. Rates are likely to vary depending on the type of clinical setting, such as child and adolescent psychiatry, pediatric neurology, or general pediatrics.

Co-occurrence of psychiatric disorders and TS may be a function of several conditions: 1) a known genetically linked association with TS, such as has been established with Obsessive Compulsive Disorder (OCD), 2) independently occurring conditions without an established genetic link, for example, generalized anxiety disorder, and 3) a secondary consequence of having TS, such as major depressive disorder[4]. It is also possible that an interaction between the underlying genetically determined neurobiology and stressful environmental factors can render an individual with TS more likely to have comorbid conditions, particularly mood or anxiety disorders[5].

Attention Deficit Hyperactivity Disorder (ADHD) and OCD are the two most commonly observed co-occurring psychiatric disorders in clinically referred youth with TS. ADHD symptoms develop before the age of 7 and thus often predate the development of tics, while OCD symptoms typically develop following the onset of tics. Most importantly, co-occurring ADHD and OCD typically interfere more often with patients' overall functioning and academic and work performance than do the tics themselves. For example, a recent measure of functional impairment in youth with TS conducted by Storch and colleagues found that non-tic related problems caused more dysfunction than the presence of tics themselves, most often as a result of either ADHD or OCD symptoms[6].

Comorbid psychiatric disorder outcomes are generally semi-independent of tic outcomes. Many of these disorders, such as ADHD and OCD, are more likely than tics to persist into adulthood, imposing functional impairment. Given the frequency with which comorbid conditions occur and the potential associated impairment, they must be anticipated, identified and optimally treated.

IMPACT AND EVALUATION OF ASSOCIATED PSYCHIATRIC CONDITIONS

Psychiatric conditions observed in patients with TS may have a variable impact, depending on the type, number and severity of disorders that are present. Given that most individuals referred for evaluation and treatment of TS will have at least one, if not multiple, psychiatric disorders, it is important to comprehensively evaluate each patient for the presence of these disorders and assesses his or her respective distress and/or impairment.

Comprehensive evaluation should always include a formal assessment of the psychiatric disorders commonly observed with the tic disorders, including ADHD and other disruptive behavior disorders, OCD, other anxiety disorders, and mood disorders. Structured or semi-structured diagnostic interviews, such as the Diagnostic Interview Schedule for Children or the Children's Schedule for Affective Disorders and Schizophrenia provide information that can lead to formal diagnoses consistent with the <u>Diagnostic and Statistical Manual, Fourth Edition</u>[7]. These instruments systematically inquire about all relevant psychiatric disorders including current and lifetime history of symptoms and level of severity, thus ensuring that co-occurring disorders are identified.

Since co-occurring psychiatric disorders may impact the patient's clinical presentation, assessment of their severity contributes to the overall illness picture. Standardized rating instruments can provide quantitative measures of tic severity, such as number, frequency, intensity, complexity and interference, and tic-related impairment.

The Yale-Global Tic Severity Scale and the Tourette syndrome Symptom List rate tics, compulsions, and other associated features[8]. Specific rating scales for OCD[9], ADHD, anxiety and mood disorders are also available and recommended. Quantitative measures of non-tic symptoms can be helpful in the prioritization of target symptoms for treatment.

Attention Deficit Hyperactivity Disorder (ADHD)

ADHD is the most common psychiatric condition associated with TS. ADHD is characterized by an enduring pattern of developmentally inappropriate inattention and/or hyperactivity and impulsive behavior. Onset of symptoms occurs before age 7. In order to meet criteria for the full disorder, some impairment from the symptoms must be present in at least two settings, most often home and school. Co-occurring TS and ADHD are often associated with academic difficulties, peer rejection, family conflict, and disruptive behaviors such as oppositional defiant behavior, aggression, low frustration tolerance, and poor compliance with treatment.

There is a bidirectional relationship between tics and ADHD; 50 to 75% of clinically referred children and adolescents with TS meet criteria for ADHD, and 10% to about a third of ADHD patients also meet criteria for a tic disorder[10-16]. The nature of the relationship between ADHD and TS is not firmly established. There are several theories addressing the overlap of TS and ADHD. Some investigators have suggested that there is a genetic relationship and that dysregulation of dopamine neurotransmitter function is a component of an underlying mechanism for both disorders[16]. Other investigators have postulated that there are two types of ADHD in patients and families with TS: one type precedes TS and is genetically independent, and the other follows the TS and is part of the syndrome[17]. It is also possible that the disorders are completely unrelated and they co-occur due to ascertainment bias; that is, patients evaluated in a specialized clinic are likely to have both more severe symptoms and co-occurring disorders than those identified in community samples. Regardless of underlying cause, the presence of ADHD predicts greater functional impairment than that associated with tic disorders alone[21]. Comorbid ADHD tends to be more persistent than tics; both in children and adults, and the tics have little impact on subsequent adult ADHD outcome[22-23].

Learning and academic problems are common in children with TS; in a database of 5,450 patients with TS, 1,235 (22.7%) had learning disabilities[18]. Young patients with TS may experience problems with executive function, such as planning, persistence, organizational skills, and social problem solving[19]. Patients with TS have also been shown to have difficulties with procedural learning, fine motor control, motor inhibition, nonverbal memory, and visual motor integration. In addition, handwriting is often poor. However, the presence of cognitive deficits in children and adults with TS are highly variable across studies; most studies have documented that the learning and executive function deficits result from the ADHD, and not TS alone. Among children with TS and comorbid ADHD, it is the ADHD that is most likely to impose disability burden. Notably, some studies have reported that children with TS but without ADHD have better motor coordination and intellectual abilities than those with ADHD alone or ADHD plus TS[20]. It is important to keep in mind that when untreated children with ADHD or OCD are assessed, the test results may not reflect the child's full capabilities and could lead to an inaccurate clinical picture.

Given the high rates of co-occurrence, systematic assessment of ADHD symptoms is necessary in all clinically referred patients with TS. Validated and normed rating instruments, such as the Swanson, Nelson and Pelham SNAP, DuPaul's ADHD-Rating Scale, or the Conners Check List can be helpful in evaluation of level of severity of ADHD symptoms[24-27]. All of these instruments have both parent and teacher report versions.

Treatment should be considered in all patients with ADHD who have impairment in academic, social or behavioral function, regardless of presence of tics. A multifaceted approach is recommended, including medication, educational assessment and services, individual therapy/ coaching, and in younger patients, parent-child interaction therapy[28]. Recent studies have suggested that stimulants, the most effective medication treatment for ADHD symptoms in patients without tics, can be used judiciously in TS patients. Despite older case reports and current labeling warnings, there is no recent scientific evidence of increased tics in patients with tic disorders and ADHD taking stimulants[29-32]. There are no controlled studies published to date of the longer acting stimulant delivery systems, although they are often well tolerated anecdotally. It is possible that avoidance of the "peaks and valleys" in blood levels of the longer acting agents reduces the likelihood of tic exacerbation from day to day.

For patients who cannot tolerate stimulants, treatment with an alpha adrenergic agonist such as guanfacine or clonidine may be helpful for ADHD symptoms, such as impulsivity and motor restlessness, as well as the tics[33-35]. In addition, atomoxetine may also be helpful; a recent study demonstrated that children with ADHD and tics experienced no increase in tics on atomoxetine compared to those on a placebo, and in fact, that tics improved relative to placebo[36].

Educational assessment and supportive services are a core component of treatment of the child with ADHD and TS. Comprehensive behavioral intervention for tics (habit reversal therapy) may be useful;

a combination of stimulant treatment and habit reversal therapy may also be helpful for children with co-occurring tics and ADHD.

Anxiety and Mood Disorders

Anxiety and mood disorders observed in clinically referred youth with TS may result from several factors. It is possible that there may be an etiologic association between TS and emotional disorders at a rate higher than chance. Recently developed neurobiological models support theoretical relationships between movement and emotion, primarily through contiguous pathways in the basal ganglia, thalamus, and cortex[37-41].

In addition, living with a chronic and potentially socially impairing illness may result in emotional distress and loss of self-esteem. Repeated experiences of demoralization, sadness, social anxiety and inhibition related to having TS could render the child more vulnerable to acute or chronic disorders with mixed anxiety and/or depressive features. Some studies have reported that children with TS have difficulty with peer relations and social skills which could lead to anxiety and depression[42].

Whatever the cause, in clinical settings, emotional symptoms are very common, and may often be more problematic to the patient than the tics. These symptoms and disorders need to be comprehensively identified, and differentiated from tics, since they require specific intervention and treatment. Reduction in tic severity may be useful but not sufficient to fully address symptoms of anxiety or depression in people with TS.

Obsessive Compulsive Disorder (OCD)

OCD is characterized by the occurrence of either obsessions, which are recurrent, intense, intrusive ideas, thoughts, impulses, or images; or compulsions, which are repetitive behaviors or mental acts intended to prevent or reduce anxiety or distress. There appears to be a bi-directional relationship between TS and OCD in most patient groups. Twenty to 40% of TS patients have been reported to meet full criteria for OCD, and up to 90% have been reported to have developing symptoms [36, 43-45]. Patients with OCD have about a 7% lifetime risk of developing TS and 20% risk of developing tics[46, 69].

Genetic studies have firmly established the link between TS and OCD; first degree (close) relatives of patients with TS have an increased risk for OCD, even if they do not have a tic disorder. Female first degree relatives of TS probands appear to have a higher risk for OCD, whereas male relatives have an increased risk for tic disorders[47-49].

TS and OCD share many common features, including a waxing and waning course, repetitive behaviors, complex movements or rituals, preoccupation with sexual and aggressive themes, and partially voluntary suppression of symptoms with subsequent buildup of inner tension. In addition, previous studies have suggested that patients with TS plus OCD have higher levels of disability than those without comorbid OCD[41, 50-52].

Patients with TS are reported to have OCD symptoms that differ in phenomenology from patients with OCD without tic disorders. Patients with TS plus OCD/obsessive compulsive behavior often describe sensory and motor symptoms associated with their repetitive behaviors, whereas patients with OCD without TS tend to experience more cognitive/affective symptoms associated with their repetitive behaviors[53]. Patients with TS and OCD often describe a need or feeling to get things "just right," and behaviors are repeated in order to achieve a feeling of symmetry balance or exactness in touch or appearance. In contrast, patients with OCD without TS, contamination or illness concerns tend to be more predominant. The distinctions may imply a different cause (i.e., TS vs. non-TS OCD), lifetime course and management strategy[54].

While obsessive compulsive behavior/OCD may emerge at any point during childhood and up through adolescence, symptoms usually peak roughly 2 years after tic symptoms peak, or may emerge after tics subside. A recent study of the course of TS in 46 patients who were evaluated initially at mean age 11, and followed up at mean age 19, indicated that about 40% reported at least moderate OCD symptoms at least once over the course of their disorder. In this study, worst ever OCD symptoms occurred approximately 2 years later than worst ever tic symptoms.

Systematic quantitative assessment of OCD symptoms is recommended with the Children's Yale Brown Obsessive Compulsive Scale. This is administered by a clinician in a semi-structured interview, and includes an inventory of obsessions and compulsions, and quantitative assessment of time occupied, interference, distress, resistance and degree of control over obsessions and compulsions[9,55]. There is considerable overlap in appearance, and to some degree, classification, in complex motor tics and compulsions; both types of symptoms manifest as repetitive, apparently purposeful behaviors involving multiple muscle groups. For example, repetitive touching/ tapping a surface or corners may represent either a compulsion or complex motor tic. Assessment of the preceding, or premonitory experience may be helpful in differentiation of the behavior[56].

Treatment of OCD is indicated if the symptoms are causing distress and/or impairment to the child. A multifaceted treatment approach is generally recommended, which includes both psychosocial intervention and medication. For psychosocial treatment, exposure and response prevention, a form of cognitive behavioral treatment, has been shown to be effective in children and adolescents with OCD. Medication is also an option; there are several controlled trials of selective serotonin reuptake inhibitors in youth with OCD[57-59]. As most treatment studies have excluded subjects with TS and OCD, there is little data as to whether CBT and SSRIs are effective for OCD symptoms observed in people with TS.

Non-OCD Anxiety Disorders

Anxiety symptoms are common in children, as are anxiety disorders, which are characterized by excessive and unrealistic worry or fear. Common anxiety disorders in children include separation anxiety, in which fear of separation from attachment figures predominates, generalized anxiety, in which excessive, unrealistic worry about performance and the future predominates, and social anxiety disorder, in which fear of embarrassment or excessive shyness predominate. Panic disorder is characterized by sudden onset of anxiety attacks without apparent cause. Panic disorder, with or without agoraphobia, a fear of going outside, is less common in children and adolescents. Co-occurring anxiety disorders are frequently observed in clinically referred youth (30-40%) and adults with TS[1, 60].

Interestingly, while co-occurrence with OCD has long been recognized as associated with more severe TS[41, 57, 61-63], less appreciated is the important role of non-OCD anxiety disorders in TS patients. Non-OCD anxiety disorders are likely more frequent in TS patients than in the general population, and encompass a wide range of conditions that can also be associated with significant reduction in quality of life and impairment[1, 49, 64-68].

In a clinical sample of 190 children with TS, non-OCD anxiety disorders, including panic disorder, agoraphobia, separation anxiety disorder, and overanxious disorder, and especially separation anxiety disorder, were highly associated with tic severity. In this study, subjects were divided into mild/moderate and severe tic severity groups. Psychiatric comorbidity was overwhelmingly present irrespective of tic severity status (94.8% for mild/moderate TS and 100% for severe TS). With the exception of social and simple phobia, all other anxiety disorders were significantly over-represented among TS subjects. It is noteworthy that separation anxiety disorder was the disorder that most robustly predicted high tic severity, even when controlling for the presence of OCD or other anxiety disorders. These findings reveal the importance of non-OCD anxiety disorders as risk factors for tic severity in children with TS. Since in this sample patients with OCD had a greater likelihood of also having non-OCD anxiety disorders, it is possible that OCD was a modulator of tic severity. Although OCD is frequently comorbid with other anxiety disorders[69-70], these findings suggest specific associations between tic severity and non-OCD anxiety disorders that are not accounted for by the presence of OCD alone.

Evidence that anxiety may contribute to tic severity is supported in the frequent worsening of tics that occur in children with TS before they return to school, and in the tic reducing effects of the high potency benzodiazepine anxiolytic clonazepam[71-72]. The alpha—adrenergic agonist drugs guanfacine and clonidine may also reduce tics through their potential anxiety-reducing effects[73-78]. Considering that antipsychotics have been reported to be associated with separation anxiety and school refusal syndromes in TS patients[79-81], it is possible that antipsychotics themselves may contribute to the development of anxiety. In addition, it is also possible that anxiety-associated hyper-arousal could result in central nervous system (CNS) noradrenergic spikes that may disrupt or hyper-sensitize the pathways involved in TS[36,82-85]. Finally, findings of reduced gamma-aminobutyric acid, the primary CNS inhibitory neurotransmitter chemical, in the CNS pathways involved in TS, support the hypothesis of increased vulnerability to anxiety in TS patients.

Comprehensive assessment of anxiety disorders should include the use of standardized rating scales, including self-reports such as the Multidimensional Anxiety Scale for Children, or Screen for Child Anxiety Related Emotional Disorders[86-87].

Treatment of anxiety disorders in patients with TS requires a comprehensive assessment of both type and level of anxiety severity. Often, in children, as anxiety disorders co-occur and cluster together, careful evaluation is indicated. For anxiety disorders with mild to moderate symptoms, cognitive behavioral treatment is usually the first approach. For patients with more severe anxiety, significant distress or functional impairment, medication treatment is usually recommended. There are several controlled studies of the selective serotonin reuptake inhibitors in pediatric patients with anxiety but without tics, which also may be used for youth with TS[88-89]. Clonazepam, an anti-anxiety medication which works through the gamma-aminobutyric acid neurotransmitter system, may be helpful for short term treatment of anxiety symptoms in patients with TS. Although controlled studies are lacking, it is often reported clinically that treatment of anxiety first can lead to reduction of tics secondarily.

Mood Disorders

Mood disorders in children are characterized by symptoms of depressed or irritable mood and loss of interest in pleasurable activities lasting for at least two weeks. Mood symptoms are common in children and adolescents. Mood disorders, including major depression and bipolar disorder, have been described frequently in clinically referred TS patients[90-93]. Whether these emotional disorders are related to the underlying neurobiology of TS, occur independently of the risk for TS, or are secondary to the demoralization and/or impairment related to having a chronic illness remains to be clarified.

Both children and adults with TS are at risk for mood disorders[1, 49, 90, 95], and, similar to the population at large, etiology is multi-factorial. It is not entirely clear whether patients with TS are at greater risk for mood disorders than other patients with chronic illness. A recent study suggests that older adolescents with TS are at risk for major depression[91]. Tic severity may or may not correlate with depression, but adults with TS with coprolalia (involuntary uttering of obscenities) report higher depressive symptoms than those without coprolalia[94].

Comorbid ADHD and OCD also independently increase the risk for depression; in addition, tic suppressing antipsychotic medications prescribed to children and adults can increase the risk.

Bipolar disorder has also been reported as occurring in clinical samples of youth and adults with TS. In a study of 156 clinically referred youth with TS, high lifetime rates of mood disorders were reported, as was a significant association between mood disorders and overall illness related impairment, measured by need for psychiatric hospitalization. Twelve percent of the 156 children and adolescents with TS, required psychiatric hospitalization. While tic severity was a marginally significant predictor of hospitalization, major depression and bipolar disorder were robust predictors of psychiatric hospitalization, even after adjusting for all other variables[96-97].

The finding of a high prevalence rate for bipolar disorder in children with severe tics is both novel and intriguing. Although the diagnosis of childhood bipolar disorder remains controversial, recent studies document that it can be reliably made when using structured diagnostic interview procedures[98].

Evaluation of mood symptoms in youth with TS should include standardized rating scales including self-reports, such as the Children's Depression Inventory, and/or clinician administered instrument such as the Children's Depression Rating Scale for major depression, and the Young Mania Rating Scale in bipolar disorder[99-101].

For treatment of mild depression, cognitive behavioral, interpersonal or individual supportive therapy is recommended. For moderate to severe symptoms, treatment with medication is often necessary, and there is established evidence for the efficacy of SSRIs in children and adolescents[102]. A diagnosis of bipolar disorder is almost always an indication for medication. There are several medications formally approved for treatment of bipolar disorder in older children/adolescents, including aripiprazole, risperidone, quetiapine, olanzapine, and lithium. Controlled studies of risperidone have also supported its use in the treatment of TS; open studies of aripiprazole have also suggested benefit in TS, so these medications would be recommended as first line options for comorbid bipolar disorder and TS.

OTHER PSYCHIATRIC CONDITIONS

Substance Use Disorders

Substance abuse and dependence occur commonly in many psychiatric disorders among affected adolescents and adults. There is little data regarding the prevalence of substance use disorders in adolescents with TS, but there is some data to suggest that adults with TS may be more likely to have problems in this area[103]. Alcohol abuse is reported in 30% of adults with TS. TS patients often report a marked reduction in premonitory urges and tics with alcohol consumption[104]. Those who use tobacco often report its beneficial effect in tic reduction, although it is unclear if the true benefit comes as direct tic reduction or reduction of mood or anxiety symptoms. Transdermal nicotine has been studied in treatment of TS[105-107].

GENERAL TREATMENT CONSIDERATIONS OF PSYCHIATRIC CONDITIONS

For patients with clinically significant co-occurring behavioral and emotional symptoms or disorders, treatment should be tailored to the specific diagnosis or symptoms of most concern. Education regarding the nature of the psychiatric disorder, parent guidance, referral to support groups, and ongoing monitoring are essential for all patients and their families. Children with mild symptoms and/or mild tics may need only supportive monitoring, or brief, supportive therapy. Identification and treatment of co-occurring conditions may result in secondary tic reduction, suggesting co-occurring conditions may be the most important initial target of treatment rather than tics.

Non-medication treatments of the psychiatric disorders associated with TS are generally recommended as the first approach for patients with mild to moderate symptoms. The most substantial evidence base points to the efficacy of cognitive behavioral treatments, such as exposure and response prevention for OCD, and interpersonal therapy for mood disorders.

Clinically referred youth with TS may often meet criteria for several co-occurring psychiatric disorders of clinical concern, such as ADHD, OCD and major depression. In such cases, patients may require the simultaneous use of more than one treatment. Unlike in other psychiatric disorders in youth not associated with tics, in which multi-modal treatment has been investigated, such as Pediatric OCD Treatment Study and Treatment for Adolescents with Depression Study, there are no multimodal treatment studies of TS and co-occurring disorders to date[108-109].

In many cases, patients may require simultaneous use of more than one medication to treat both tics and emotional or behavioral symptoms. This approach, described as "targeted combined pharmacotherapy," involves the careful, judicious use of more than one medication, simultaneously, for two different, but co-occurring disorders. The combined use of clonidine and methylphenidate, for example, was investigated recently in the treatment of tics and ADHD[31]. This approach demonstrated that both disorders could be treated independently and simultaneously, carefully targeting symptoms of each disorder. Results showed not only independent and additive efficacy in reduction of tics and ADHD symptoms, but that adverse effects were minimal and in this combination, neutralized one another. That said, targeted combined pharmacotherapy should be carefully monitored and periodically re-evaluated, since both tics and emotional or behavioral symptoms wax and wane.

Medication trials should be initiated by the introduction of one medication at a time, exploiting the full benefit of one medication before targeted combined pharmacotherapy is necessary. The primary goal of treatment should be an adequate trial of each agent in terms of dosage and duration. For the majority of patients, medication should be initiated at a low (usually sub-therapeutic) dose and gradually increased upward. Therapeutic effects and adverse effects should be closely monitored, especially when more than one agent is administered simultaneously. When targeted combined pharmacotherapy is used, adverse effects of drug interactions are more likely. The primary goal of treatment should be an adequate trial of each agent in terms of dosage and duration.

References

1. Robertson, M.M., Channon, S., Baker, J. & Flynn, D. (1993) The psychopathology of Gilles de la Tourette's syndrome. A controlled study. *Br J Psychiatry* **162,** 114-117.
2. Coffey,B.,Miguel,E.,Biederman,J.,Baer,L.,Rauch,S.,O'Sullivan, R., Savage, C., Phillips, K., Borgman, A., Green-Leibovitz, M., Moore, E., Park, K. & Jenike, M. (1998) Tourette's Disorder with and without Obsessive Compulsive Disorder in Adults: Are they Different? *J Nerv Ment Dis* **186,** 201-215.
3. Robertson, M.M. (2000) Tourette Syndrome, associated conditions and the complexities of treatment. *Brain* **123,** 425-462.
4. Gaze, C., Kepley, H.O. & Walkup, J.T. (2006) Co-occurring Psychiatric Disorders in Children and Adolescents With Tourette Syndrome. *J Child Neurol* **21,** 657-664.
5. Lin, H., Katsovich, L., Ghebremichael, M., Findley, D.B., Grantz, H., Lombroso, P.J., King, R.A., Zhang, H. & Leckman, J.F. (2007) Psychosocial stress predicts future symptom severities in children and adolescents with Tourette syndrome and/or obsessive-compulsive disorder. *J Child Psychol Psychiatry* **48,** 157-166.
6. Storch, E.A., Lack, C.W., Simons, L.E., Goodman, W.K., Murphy, T.K. & Geffken, G.R. (2007) A Measure of Functional Impairment in Youth with Tourette's Syndrome. *J Pediatr Psychol* **32,** 950-959.
7. Association AP. (1994) *Diagnostic and Statistical Manual of Mental Disorders, Fourth Edition.* American Psychiatric Press, Inc, Washington, D.C.
8. Leckman, J.F., Riddle, M.A., Hardin, M.T., Ort, S.I., Swartz, K.L., Stevenson, J. & Cohen, D.J. (1989) The Yale Global Tic Severity Scale: Initial testing of a clinician-rated scale of tic severity. *J Am Acad Child Adolesc Psychiatry* **28,** 566-573.
9. Goodman, W.K., Price, L.H., Rasmussen, S.A., Mazure, C., Delgado, P., Heninger, G.R. & Charney, D.S. (1989a) The Yale-Brown Obsessive Compulsive Scale (YBOCS) Part II: Validity. *Arch Gen Psychiatry* **46,** 1012-1016.

10. Comings, D.E. & Comings, B.G. (1987) A controlled study of Tourette syndrome. IV. Obsessions, compulsions, and schizoid behaviors. *Am J Hum Genet* **41,** 782-803.

11. Comings, D. (1990) 'ADHD in Tourette syndrome', in *Tourette Syndrome and Human Behavior*, (D. Comings, ed.) pp.99-104 Hope Press, Duarte, CA.

12. Kadesjö, B. & Gillberg, C. (2001) The comorbidity of ADHD in the general population of Swedish school-age children. *J Child Psychol Psychiatry* **42,** 487-492.

13. MTA Cooperative Group. (1999) A 14-month randomized clinical trial of treatment strategies for attention-deficit/hyperactivity disorder. Multimodal Treatment Study of Children with ADHD. *Arch Gen Psychiatry* **56,** 1073-1086.

14. Shapiro, A. (1988a) Epidemiology in *Gilles de la Tourette Syndrome*, (Shapiro, A., Shapiro, E., Young, J. G. & Feinberg, T. eds.) pp. 45-50 Raven Press, NY.

15. Shapiro, A. (1988b) Signs, Symptoms, and Clinical Course in *Gilles de la Tourette Syndrome*, (Shapiro, A., Shapiro, E., Young, J. G. & Feinberg, T. eds) pp.169-193 Raven Press, NY.

16. Spencer, T., Biederman, J., Harding, M., Wilens, T. & Faraone, S. (1995) The Relationship between Tic Disorders and Tourette's Syndrome Revisited. *J Am Acad Child Adolesc Psychiatry* **34,** 1133-1139.

17. Pauls, D.L., Leckman, J.F. & Cohen, D.J. (1993) Familial Relationship between Gilles de la Tourette's Syndrome, Attention Deficit Disorder, Learning Disabilities, Speech Disorders, and Stuttering. *J Am Acad Child Adolesc Psychiatry* **32,** 1044-1050.

18. Burd, L., Freeman, R.D., Klug, M.G. & Kerbeshian, J. (2005) Tourette syndrome and learning disabilities. *BMC Pediatr* **5,** 34.

19. Lavoie, M.E., Thibault, G., Stip, E. & O'Connor, K.P. (2007) Memory and executive functions in adults with Gilles de la Tourette syndrome and chronic tic disorder. *Cogn Neuropsychiatry* **12,** 165-181.

20. Denckla, M.B. (2006) Attention deficit hyperactivity disorder: the childhood co-morbidity that most influences the disability burden in Tourette syndrome. *Adv Neurol* **99,** 17-21.

21. Sukhodolsky, D.G., Scahill, S., Zhang, H., Peterson, B.S., King, R.A., Lombroso, P.J., Katsovich, L., Findley, D. & Leckman, J.F.

(2003) Disruptive Behavior in Children with Tourette's Syndrome: Association with ADHD Comorbidity, Tic Severity, and Functional Impairment. *J Am Acad of Child Adolesc Psychiatry* **42,** 98-105.

22. Spencer, T., Biederman, J., Coffey, B., Geller, D., Wilens, T. & Faraone, S. (1999) The 4-Year Course of Tic Disorders in Boys with Attention-Deficit/Hyperactivity Disorder. *Arch Gen Psychiatry* **56,** 842-847.

23. Spencer, T.J., Biederman, J., Stephen, F., Mick, E., Coffey, B., Geller, D., Kagan, J., Bearman, S.K. & Wilens, T. (2001) Impact of Tic Disorders on ADHD Outcome Across the Life Cycle: Findings From a Large Group of Adults With and Without ADHD. *Am J Psychiatry* **158,** 611-617.

24. DuPaul, G.J., Power, T.J., Anastopoulos, A.D. & Reid, R. (1998) ADHD Rating Scale-IV: Checklists, Norms, and Clinical Interpretation.

25. Loney, J. & Milich, R. (1982) Hyperactivity, inattention, and aggression in clinical practice. *Adv Beh Pediatr* **2,** 113–147.

26. Pelham, W.E., Milich, R., Murphy, D.A. & Murphy, H.A. (1989) Normative data on the IOWA Conners teacher rating scale. *J Clin Child Psychology* **18,** 259–262.

27. Swanson, J.M. (1992) *School Based Assessments and Interventions for ADD Students*. K.C. Publishing, Irvine, CA.

28. Rube, D. & Reddy, D.P. (2006) Attention Deficit Hyperactivity Disorder, in *Clin Child Psychiatry*, Second Edition (Klykylo, W.M., and Kay, J.L. eds.), John Wiley & Sons, Ltd.

29. Gadow, K.D., Sverd, J., Nolan, E.E., Sprafkin, J. & Schneider, J. (2007) Immediate-Release Menthylphenidate for ADHD in Children With Comorbid Chronic Multiple Tic Disorder. *J Am Acad Child Adolesc Psychiatry* **46,** 840-848.

30. Gadow, K.D., Nolan, E.E. & Sverd, J. (1992) Methylphenidate in hyperactive boys with comorbid tic disorder: II. Short-term behavioral effects in school settings. *J Am Acad Adolesc Psychiatry* **31,** 462-471.

31. Tourette Syndrome Study Group (TSSG): Treatment of ADHD in children with tics: A randomized controlled trial. (2002) *Neurology* **58,** 527–536.

32. Lyon, G.J., Samar, S.M., Conelea, C., Trujillo, M.R., Lipinski, C.M., Bauer, C.C., Brandt, B.C., Kemp, J.J., Lawrence, Z.E., Howard,

J., Castellanos, F.X., Woods, D. & Coffey, B.J. (2010) Testing Tic Suppression: Comparing the Effects of Dexmethylphenidate to No Medication in Children and Adolescents with Attention-Deficit/ Hyperactivity Disorder and Tourette's Disorder. *J Child and Adolesc Psychopharmacol* **20**, 283-289.

33. Chappell, P.B., Riddle, M.A., Scahill, L., Lynch, K.A., Schultz, R., Arnsten, A., Leckman, J.F. & Cohen, D.J. (1995) Guanfacine Treatment of Comorbid Attention-Deficit Hyperactivity Disorder and Tourette's Syndrome: Preliminary Clinical Experience. *J Am Acad Child Adolesc Psychiatry* **34**, 1140-1146.

34. Scahill, L., Chappell, P.B., Kim, Y.S., Schultz, R.T., Katsovich, L., Shepherd, E., Arnsten, A.F.T., Cohen, D.J. & Leckman, J.F. (2001) A Placebo-Controlled Study of Guanfacine in the Treatment of Children with Tic Disorders and Attention Deficit Hyperactivity Disorder. *Am J Psychiatry* **158**, 1067-1074.

35. Steingard, R., Biederman, J., Spencer, T., Wilens, T. & Gonzalez, A. (1993) Comparison of Clonidine Response in the Treatment of Attention-Deficit Hyperactivity Disorder with and without Comorbid Tic Disorders. *J Am Acad Child Adolesc Psychiatry* **32**, 350-353.

36. Allen, A.J., Kurlan, R.M., Gilbert, D.L., Coffey, B.J., Linder, S.L., Lewis, D.W., Winner, P.K., Dunn, D.W., Dure, L.S., Sallee, F.R., Milton, D.R., Mintz, M.I., Ricardi, R.K., Erenberg, G., Layton, L.L., Feldman, P.D., Kelsey, D.K. & Spencer, T.J. (2005) Atomoxetine treatment in children and adolescents with ADHD and comorbid tic disorders. *Neurology* **65**, 1941-1949.

37. Cohen, D.J., Friedhoff, A.J. & Leckman, J.F., Chase, T.N. (1992) Tourette syndrome. Extending basic research to clinical care. [Review]. *Adv Neurol* **58**, 341-362.

38. Cohen, D.J. & Leckman, J.F. (1994) Developmental psychopathology and neurobiology of Tourette's syndrome. [Review]. *J Am Acad Child Adolesc Psychiatry* **33**, 2-15.

39. Wolf, S.J., Douglas, Knable, M., Gorey J., Lee, K.S., Hyde, T., Coppola, R. & Weinberger, D. (1996) Tourette Syndrome: Prediction of Phenotypic Variation in Monozygotic Twins by Caudate Nucleus D2 Receptor Binding. *Science* **273(5279)**, 1225-1227.

40. Singer, H.S., Walkup, J.T. (1991) Tourette syndrome and other tic disorders. Diagnosis, pathophysiology, and treatment. [Review]. *Medicine* **70,** 15-32.

41. Demeter, S. (1992) Structural imaging in Tourette syndrome. [Review]. *Adv Neurol* **58,** 201-206.

42. Stokes, A., Bawden, H.N., Camfield, P.R., Backman, J.E. & Dooley, J.M. (1991) Peer problems in Tourette's disorder. *Pediatrics* **87,** 936-942.

43. Comings, D.E. & Comings, B.G. (1987) A controlled study of Tourette syndrome. I. Attention-deficit disorders, and school problems. *Am J Hum Genet* **41,** 701-741.

44. Frankel, M., Cummings, J.L., Robertson, M.M., Trimble, M.R., Hill, M.A. & Benson, D.F. (1986) Obsessions and compulsions in Gilles de la Tourette's syndrome. *Neurology* **36,** 378-382.

45. Grad, L.R., Pelcovits, D., Olson, M., Matthews, M. & Grad, G. (1987) Obsessive-Compulsive Symptomatology in children with Tourette's Syndrome. *Am Acad Child Adolesc Psychiatry* **26,** 69-73.

46. Swedo, S., Rapoport, J., Leonard, H., Lenane, M., & Cheslow, D. (1989) Obsessive Compulsive Disorder in children and adolescents. *Arch Gen Psychiatry* **46,** 335.

47. Pauls, D.L., Hurst, C.R, Kruger, S.D., Leckman, J.F., Kidd, K.K. & Cohen, D.J. (1986) Gilles de la Tourette's syndrome and attention deficit disorder with hyperactivity. Evidence against a genetic relationship. *Arch Gen Psychiatry* **43,** 1177-1179.

48. Pauls, D.L., Raymond, C.L., Stevenson, J.M. & Leckman, J.F. (1991) A family study of Gilles de la Tourette syndrome. *Am J Hum Genet* **48,** 154-163.

49. Pauls, D.L. (1992) The genetics of obsessive compulsive disorder and Gilles de la Tourette's syndrome. [Review]. *Psychiatr Clin North Am* **15,** 759-766.

50. Pitman, R.K., Green, R.C., Jenike, M.A. & Mesulam, M.M. (1987) Clinical comparison of Tourette's disorder and obsessive-compulsive disorder. *Am J Psychiatry* **144,** 1166-1171.

51. Bruun, R.D. & Budman, C.L. (1997) The course and prognosis of Tourette Syndrome. *Neurol Clin* **15,** 291-298.

52. Leonard, H.L., Swedo, S.E., Rapoport, J.L., Rickler, K.C., Topol, D., Lee, S. & Rettew, D. (1992) Tourette syndrome and obsessive-compulsive disorder. [Review]. *Adv Neurol* **58**, 83-93.

53. Miguel, E.C., Rosario-Campos, M.C., Prado, H.S., Valle, R., Rauch, S.L., Coffey, B.J., Baer, L., Savage, C.R., O'Sullivan, R.L., Jenicke, M.A. & Leckman, J.F. (2000) Sensory phenomena in obsessive-compulsive disorder and Tourette's disorder. *J Clin Psychiatry* **61**, 150-157.

54. Leckman, J.F., Walke, D.E., Goodman, W.K., Pauls, D.L. & Cohen, D.J. "Just right" perceptions associated with compulsive behavior in Tourette's syndrome. *Am J Psychiatry* **151**, 675-680.

55. Goodman, W.K., Price, L H., Rasmussen, S.A., Mazure, C., Delgado, P., Heninger, G.R. & Charney, D.S. (1989b) The Yale-Brown Obsessive Compulsive Scale (YBOCS) Part I: Development, use and reliability. *Arch Gen Psychiatry* **46**, 1006-1011.

56. Miguel, E.C., Coffey, B.J., Baer, L., Savage, C., Rauch, S.L. & Jenike, M.A. 'Phenomenology of intentional repetitive behaviors in obsessive compulsive disorder and Tourette's disorder', *J Clin Psychiatry* **56**, 246-255.

57. Riddle, M.A., Hardin, M.T., King, R., Scahill, L. & Woolston, J.L. (1990) 'Fluoxetine treatment of children and adolescents with Tourette's and obsessive compulsive disorders: preliminary clinical experience', *J Am Acad Child Adolesc Psychiatry* **29**, 45-48.

58. Kurlan, R., Como, P.G., Deeley, C., McDermott, M. & McDermott, M.P. (1993) A pilot controlled study of fluoxetine for obsessive-compulsive symptoms in children with Tourette's syndrome. *Clin Neuropharmacol* **16**, 167-172.

59. Pediatric OCD Treatment Study (POTS) Team, 2004 Pediatric OCD Treatment Study (POTS) Team. (2004) Cognitive-behavior therapy, sertraline, and their combination for children and adolescents with obsessive-compulsive disorder: the Pediatric OCD Treatment Study (POTS) randomized controlled trial. *JAMA* **292**, 1969–1976.

60. Coffey, B.J., Biederman, J., Geller, D., Sarin, P., Schwartz, S. & Kim, G. (2000) Distinguishing illness severity from tic severity

in children and adolescents with Tourette's Disorder. *J Am Acad Child Adolesc Psychiatry* **39,** 556-561.

61. Coffey, B.J., Biederman, J., Smoller, J., Geller, D., Sarin, P., Schwartz, S. & Kim, G. (2000) Anxiety Disorders and Tic Severity in Juveniles with Tourette's Disorder. *J Am Acad Child Adolesc Psychiatry* **39,** 562-568.

62. de Groot, C., Bornstein, R., Spetie, L. & Burriss, B.A. The Course of Tics In Tourette's Syndrome: A 5-Year Follow-up Study. *Ann Clin Psychiatry* **6,** 227-233.

63. Marcus, D.K. (2001) Tics and Its Disorders. Neurologic Clinics: *Mov Disord* **19,** 735-758.

64. Coffey, B.J., Frazier, J. & Chen, S. (1992) Comorbidity, Tourette syndrome, and anxiety disorders. [Review]. *Adv Neurol* **58,** 95-104.

65. Comings, D.E. & Comings, B.G. (1987d) A controlled study of Tourette syndrome. III: Phobias and panic attacks. *Am J Hum Genet* **41,** 761-781.

66. Nolan, E., Sverd, J., Gadow, K., Sprafkin, J. & Ezor, S. (1996) Associated psychopathology in children with both ADHD and chronic tic disorder. *J Am Acad Child Adolsesc Psychiatry* **35,** 1622-1630.

67. Cath, D., Spinhoven, P., Hoogduin, C. Landman, A.D., van Woerkman, T.C., van de Wetering, B.J. Roos, R.A. & Rooijmans, H.G. (2001) Repetitive behaviors in Tourette's Syndrome and OCD with and without tics: What are the differences? *Psychiatry Res* **101,** 171-185.

68. Rasmussen, S.A. & Eisen, J.L. (1990) Epidemiology and clinical features of obsessive-compulsive disorder in Obsessive Compulsive Disorder: Theory and Management. (Jenike M, Baer L, Minichiello W, eds.) Year Book Medical Publishers, Chicago.

69. Leonard, H., Swedo, S. & Rapoport, J. (1988) Treatment of childhood obsessive compulsive disorder with clomipramine and desmethylimipramine; a double blind crossover comparison. *Psychopharmacol Bull* **24,** 93-95.

70. Steingard, R. & Dillon-Stout, D. (1992) Tourette's syndrome and obsessive compulsive disorder. Clinical aspects [Review]. *Psychiatr Clin North Am* **15,** 849-860.

71. Goetz, C.G. (1992) Clonidine and clonazepam in Tourette syndrome. [Review]. *Adv Neurol* **58,** 245-251.

72. Borison, R.L., Ang, L., Chang, S., Dysken, M., Comaty, J.E. & Davis, J.M. (1982) New pharmacological approaches in the treatment of Tourette syndrome. *Adv Neurol* **35,** 377-382.

73. Goetz, C.G., Tanner, C.M., Wilson, R.S., Carroll, V.S., Como, P.G. & Shannon, K.M. (1987a) Clonidine and Gilles de la Tourette's syndrome: double-blind study using objective rating methods. *Ann Neurol* **21,** 307-310.

74. Bruun, R.D. (1982a) Clonidine treatment of Tourette syndrome. *Adv Neurol* **35,** 403-405.

75. Leckman, J.F., Cohen, D.J., Detlor, J., Young, J.G., Harcherik, D., & Shaywitz, B.A. (1982) Clonidine in the treatment of Tourette syndrome: A review of data. *Adv Neurol* **35,** 391-401.

76. Leckman, J.F., Hardin, M.T., Riddle, M.A., Stevenson, J., Ort, S.I. & Cohen, D.J. (1991) Clonidine treatment of Gilles de la Tourette's syndrome. *Arch Gen Psychiatry* **48,** 324-328.

77. Singer, H., Brown, J., Quaskey, S., Rosenberg, L., Mellits, D. & Denckla, M. (1995) The Treatment of Attention-Deficit Hyperactivity Disorder in Tourette's Syndrome: A Double Blind Placebo Controlled Study with Clonidine and Desipramine. *Pediatrics* **95,** 74-81.

78. Spencer, T., Biederman, J., Kerman, K., Steingard, R. & Wilens, T. Desipramine treatment of children with attention deficit hyperactivity disorder and tic disorder or Tourette's syndrome. *J Am Acad Child Adolesc Psychiatry* **32,** 354-360.

79. Bruun, R.D. (1982b) Dysphoric phenomena associated with haloperidol treatment of Tourette syndrome. *Adv Neurol* **35,** 433-436.

80. Bruun, R.D. (1988) Subtle and underrecognized side effects of neuroleptic treatment in children with Tourette's disorder. *Am J Psychiatry* **145,** 621-624.

81. Linet, L.S. (1985) Tourette syndrome, pimozide, and school phobia: The neuroleptic separation. *Am J Psychiatry* **142,** 613-615.

82. Riddle, M.A., Leckman, J.F., Anderson, G.M., Ort, S.I., Hardin, M.T, Stevenson, J. & Cohen, D.J. (1988a) Plasma MHPG: Within- and across-day stability in children and adults with Tourette's syndrome. *Biol Psychiatry* **24,** 391-398.

83. Peterson, B, Riddle, M.A., Cohen, D.J., Katz, L.D., Smith, J.C., Hardin, M.T., Leckman, J.F. (1993) Reduced basal ganglia volumes in Tourette's syndrome using three-dimensional reconstruction techniques from magnetic resonance images. *Neurology* **43**, 941-949.

84. Riddle, M.A., Leckman, J.F., Anderson, G.M., Ort, S.I., Hardin, M.T., Stevenson, J., Cohen, D.J. (1988b) Tourette's syndrome: Clinical and neurochemical correlates. *J Am Acad Child Adolesc Psychiatry* **27**, 409-412.

85. Singer, H.S., Hahn, I.H., Krowiak, E., Nelson, E. & Moran, T. (1990) Tourette's syndrome: a neurochemical analysis of postmortem cortical brain tissue. *Ann Neurol* **27**, 443-446.

86. Birmaher, B., Khetarpal, S., Brent, D., Cully, M., Balach, L., Kaufman, J. & Neer, S.M. (1997) The Screen for Child Anxiety Related Emotional Disorders (SCARED): scale construction and psychometric characteristics. *J Am Acad Child Adolesc Psychiatry* **36**, 545-553.

87. March, J.S. (1997) Multidimensional Anxiety Scale for Children: Technical manual. Multi-Health Systems. North Tonawanda, NY.

88. Siedel, L. & Walkup, J.T. (2006) Selective Serotonin Reuptake Inhibitor Use in the Treatment of the Pediatric Non-Obsessive Compulsive Disorder Anxiety Disorders. *J Child Adolesc Psychopharmacol* **16**, 171-179.

89. Birmaher, B., Axelson, D.A., Monk, K., Kalas, C., Clark, D.B., Ehmann, M., Bridge, J., Heo, J. & Brent, D.A. (2003) Fluoxetine for the Treatment of Childhood Anxiety Disorders. *J Am Acad Child Adolesc Psychiatry* **42**, 415-423.

90. Comings, B.G. & Comings, D.E. (1987) A controlled study of Tourette syndrome V. Depression and mania. *Am J Hum Genet* **41**, 804-821.

91. Gorman, D.A., Thompson, N., Plessen, K.J., Robertson, M.M., Leckman, J.F. & Peterson, B.S. (2010) Psychosocial outcome and psychiatric comorbidity in older adolescents with Tourette syndrome: controlled study. *Br J Psychiatry* **197**, 36-44.

92. Robertson, M.M. (2006) Attention deficit hyperactivity disorder, tics and Tourette's syndrome: the relationship and treatment implications. A commentary. *Eur Child Adolesc Psychiatry* **15**, 1-11.

93. Robertson, M.M., Trimble, M.R. & Lees, A.J. (1988) The psychopathology of the Gilles de la Tourette syndrome. A phenomenological analysis. *Br J Psychiatry* **152,** 383-390.

94. Cath, D., Spinhoven, P., Hoogduin, C., Landman, A.D., van Woerkman, T.C., van de Wetering, B.J., Roos, R.A. & Rooijmans, H.G. (2001) Repetitive behaviors in Tourette's Syndrome and OCD with and without tics: What are the differences? *J Psychiatry Res* **101,** 171-185.

95. Kerbeshian, J., Burd, L. & Klug, M. (1995) Comorbid Tourette's disorder and bipolar disorder: An etiologic perspective. *Am J Psychiatry* **152,** 1646-1651.

96. Berthier, M.L., J.K. & Campos, V.M. (1998) Bipolar disorder in adult patients with Tourette's syndrome: a clinical study. *Biol Psychiatry* **43,** 364-370.

97. Biederman, J., Faraone, S., Mick, E., Wozniak, J., Chen, L., Ouellette, C., Marrs, A., Moore, P., Garcia, J., Mennin, D. & Lelon, E. (1996) Attention-deficit hyperactivity disorder and juvenile mania: an overlooked comorbidity? *J Am Acad Child Adolesc Psychiatry* **35,** 997-1008.

98. Poznanski, E.O., Cook, S.C. & Carroll, B.J. (1979) A Depression Rating Scale for Children. *Pediatrics* **64,** 442-450.

99. Kovacs, M. & Beck, A.T. (1977) An Empirical Clinical Approach Towards a Definition of Childhood Depression. *Depression in Children: Diagnosis, treatment, and conceptual models.* (Schulterbrandt, J.G. & Raskin, R. eds.), Raven Press, NY.

100. Young, R.C., Biggs, J.T., Ziegler, V.E. & Meyer, D.A. (1978) A Rating Scale for Mania: Reliability, validity and sensitivity. *Br J Psychiatry* **133,** 429-435.

101. March, J.S. & TADS Team. (2007) The Treatment for Adolescents with Depression Study (TADS) – Long Term Effectiveness and Safety Outcomes. *Arch Gen Psychiatry* **64,** 1132-1143.

102. Emslie, G.J., Heiligenstein, J.H., Wagner, K.D., Hoog, S.L., Ernest, D.E., Brown, E., Nilsson, M. & Jacobson, J.G. (2002) Fluoxetine for Acute Treatment of Depression in Children and Adolescents: A Placebo-Controlled, Randomized Clinical Trial. *J Am Acad Child Adolesc Psychiatry* **41,** 1205-1215.

103. Comings, D.E. (1994) Genetic factors in substance abuse based on studies of Tourette Syndrome and ADHD probands and relatives. I. Drug abuse. *Drug Alcohol Depend* **35,** 1-16.

104. Müller-Vahl, K.R., Kolbe, H. & Dengler, R. (1997) Alcohol withdrawal and Tourette's syndrome. *Neurology* **48,** 1478-1479.

105. Mihailescu, S. & Drucker-Colin, R. (2000) Nicotine, brain nicotinic receptors, and neuropsychiatric disorders. *Arch Med Res* **31,** 131-144.

106. Sanberg, P.R., Silver, A.A., Shytle, R.D., Philipp, M.K., Cahill, D.W., Fogelson, H.M. & McConville, B.J. (1997) Nicotine for the treatment of Tourette's syndrome. *Pharmacol Ther* **74,** 21-25.

107. Silver, A.A., Shytle, R.D., Philipp, M.K., Wilkinson, B.J., McConville, B. & Sanberg, P.R. (2001) Transdermal nicotine and haloperidol in Tourette's disorder: a double-blind placebo-controlled study. *J Clin Psychiatry* **62,** 707-714.

108. Pediatric OCD Treatment Study Team [POTS]: Cognitive-behavior therapy, sertraline, and their combination with children and adolescents with Obsessive-Compulsive Disorder: The Pediatric OCD Treatment Study (POTS) randomized controlled trial. (2004) *JAMA* **292,** 1969-1976.

109. The TADS Team. (2007) The Treatment for Adolescents with Depression Study (TADS) – Long-term Effectiveness and Safety Outcomes. *Arch Gen Psychiatry* **64,** 1132-1143.

CHAPTER 4

PROBLEMS WITH ANGER, AGGRESSION, AND IMPULSE CONTROL IN TOURETTE SYNDROME

Cathy L. Budman, M.D. and Joanna Witkin, B.S.

INTRODUCTION

Aggressive symptoms, problems with anger control, and impaired impulse control are common among children and adults with TS. Data from a large international survey of TS specialists treating over 3,500 individuals with TS worldwide suggests that 37% of all TS patients have anger control problems at some point in life and 25% currently experience anger control problems[1]. Studies in the United States that evaluated clinically-referred populations of youth with TS report 25-70% experience problems with aggressive symptoms. When present, aggressive symptoms are a major cause of TS morbidity[2]. For this reason, it is essential to recognize, better understand, and appropriately treat these symptoms in people with TS.

This chapter will provide some general background on aggression, describe the phenomenology of aggressive symptoms in TS, discuss known and potential underpinnings of such symptoms, and review pharmacological and non-pharmacological treatment options for affected individuals.

BACKGROUND ON AGGRESSION

Aggression is defined as hostile or destructive behaviors or actions, and aggression can be and is adaptive in some circumstances. Among animals, several distinct types of aggression have been described, each with its particular contribution towards survival, including: predatory, intermale, territorial, maternal, and irritable aggression. *Predatory aggression* in animals refers to interspecies conflicts whereby an attacker preys on another animal, often with the goal of obtaining its next meal. *Intermale aggression* refers to aggressive behaviors among males of the same species who are competing to establish a dominance hierarchy. *Territorial aggression* refers to aggressive behaviors that are performed in an attempt to defend and protect an area or access to resources. *Maternal aggression* is characterized by aggressive behaviors that are performed to protect one's offspring or potential offspring from harm. *Irritable aggression* involves reactive, aggressive responses to undesirable environmental conditions such as excessive noise, extreme temperature, starvation or pain. Elements of each of these forms of animal aggression are also observable in humans. However, in contrast to animals, human aggression seems to have an additional cognitive component called "executive functions" that serve to oversee, integrate, and coordinate other brain activities that are central to vigilance, planning, learning, judgment, and self-control. Damage or impairment of these higher level cognitive processes can lead to increased impulsivity, poor social judgment, and problems with anger control.

Case #1—Phineas Gage

Phineas Gage, an American railroad worker in the 19th century, survived a terrible accident whereby a large iron rod was completely driven through his skull, destroying much of his brain's left frontal lobe. After his accident, Gage reportedly experienced serious adverse changes in his impulse control, personality, and behavior, effects so profound that friends saw him as "no longer Gage." His case was among the first to stimulate scientific discussion about how damage to specific regions of the brain might affect personality and behavior.

NORMAL DEVELOPMENT AND AGGRESSION

Aggressive impulses and behaviors occur in early childhood and are considered, to a point, a normal and formative part of development. "The Terrible Twos" is a phase typically observed among toddlers aged 18 through 36 months who exhibit intense outbursts of anger, displeasure, physical agitation, and opposition in response to frustration. "Temper tantrums" are aggressive behaviors most commonly observed in children ages 3-5 years that become much less frequent over time. Temper tantrums occur more often in children with a history of head trauma, seizures, bedwetting, head banging, sleep disorders, attention deficit hyperactivity disorder (ADHD), and tics. The ability to inhibit unacceptable impulses and behaviors are developmental skills that strengthen with neurological and social maturation. By the time many children enter elementary school, most are already showing capacities to tolerate frustration, delay gratification, inhibit aggressive urges, and follow rules. Temper tantrums are increasingly unusual by adolescence and early adulthood; when temper tantrums regularly occur in this age group, such behavior is generally regarded as "immature" and age—inappropriate.

Case #2—The Temper Tantrum

Jane is a 2 ½ year old whose mother just gave birth to a younger sibling two months ago. When told that she had to stop playing and put on her shoes, Jane began to scream, kicked her mother, and threw herself on the floor holding her breath until her mother feared Jane would pass out.

PATHOLOGICAL AGGRESSION

Pathological aggression is defined as aggressive behavior that is: 1) excessive in intensity, duration, and frequency; 2) inappropriate to expect social context; and 3) age-inappropriate. Aggressive behavior may be directed towards self, family, friends, strangers, animals, and/or objects. Two main types of pathologically aggressive behaviors occur in humans: proactive and reactive aggression. *Proactive aggression,* also called "non-impulsive aggression", refers to aggressive behaviors that are "premeditated" and performed to attain a specific goal. Proactive aggression has an average age of onset at 6.5 years, is associated with aggressive family role models and is characterized by low levels of physiological/emotional arousal and limited guilt or regret. Examples of proactive aggressive behaviors include: bullying, terrorism, deliberate cruelty to animals, and antisocial behaviors such as stealing or rape. *Reactive aggression*, also called "impulsive" or "non-predatory aggression", has an earlier age of onset (usually around 4.5 years), may be associated with childhood trauma or abuse, and is characterized by high levels of physiological/emotional arousal. Reactive aggression is spontaneous in nature, without obvious intention and organization aimed at achieving specific goals. It is usually triggered by an acute frustration. Explosive outbursts, "affective storms", "meltdowns", or "rage attacks" are examples of reactive aggression. Reactive aggression is much more common in clinical population than predatory aggression. In some instances, both proactive and reactive aggression can co-occur.

Case #3—Proactive Aggression: The Psychopath

Ted Bundy was a serial murderer who killed dozens of women in the 1970s by feigning injury to lure unsuspecting women to their deaths. Sometimes he deliberately put his arm in a sling to evoke sympathy and attention from his intended victims. A compulsive thief, shop lifter, and forger by the time he left high school, he became a student of psychology as a young adult and used this knowledge to grossly exploit and manipulate others.

Case #4—Reactive Aggression: "Road Rage"

Arthur is a 55 year old man who suddenly becomes extremely agitated and aggressive while driving his car. He is easily angered by other motorists whom he feels are driving poorly or "cutting him off". In addition to giving other drivers "the finger", he will sometimes open his window to shout obscenities, speed up, tail-gate, and sometimes even follow another vehicle for some distance.

PSYCHOPATHOLOGY AND AGGRESSION

Aggressive symptoms arise due to a variety of social, psychological, and biological factors, acting either alone or in combination. Pathological aggression can result from abnormal development or damage to specific areas of the brain, such as the prefrontal cortex, or amygdala and other parts of the limbic system involved in affective evaluation and regulation. Imbalances of certain neurotransmitters such as serotonin, norepinephrine, and dopamine in the prefrontal cortex, or of excitatory glutamate and inhibitory gamma-aminobutyric acid in the brain's subcortex can lead to dysregulation of angry feelings and impulses. Neuropeptides (e.g. cholecystokinin), hormones (e.g. testosterone) and immunomodulating agents (e.g. cytokines) also play a role in the regulation and expression of different types of aggressive behaviors.

Certain types of aggression appear more related to underlying genetic vulnerabilities, while other types are most directly influenced by environmental factors. In the majority of instances, aggression results from a complex interplay between an individual's underlying biology and environment.

Victims of physical, sexual or emotional abuse are at a higher risk for symptoms of pathological aggression. Poverty, poor nutrition, chaotic or excessively harsh educational or home environments, coercive or overly controlling parenting styles, as well as alcohol and/or substance abuse are also associated with increased aggressive symptoms. Aggression dysregulation symptoms can emerge as side effects from certain prescribed medications (see Table #1), over-the-counter preparations, health food supplements, dietary allergy or vitamin deficiencies. A number of medical and psychiatric conditions are associated with aggressive symptoms (see Table #2).

Table 1: Medications Side Effects Of Aggression Dysregulation

Psychoactive Medications with Possible Dysregulation Symptom Side Effects	
Zolpidem	Diphenhydramine
Benzodiazepines	Dopamine agonists
Steroids	Anticonvulsants
Psychostimulants	Antidepressants
Guanfacine	Conventional & Atypical Antipsychotics

Table 2: Psychiatric and Medical Conditions Associated with Aggressive Dysregulation

Psychiatric and Medical Conditions Associated with Aggressive Dysregualtion	
Antisocial Personality Disorder	Pain
Borderline Personality Disorder	Sleep Disorders
Major Depression	Acquired Head Injuries
Bipolar Affective Disorder	Alcohol/Substance Abuse
Schizophrenia	Dementia
Attention Deficit Hyperactivity Disorder	Delirium
Conduct Disorder	Autistic Spectrum Disorder
Oppositional Defiant Disorder	Intermittent Explosive Disorder

"Intermittent Explosive Disorder" (IED) is a condition defined by severe symptoms of reactive aggression. It is characterized by discrete episodes of failure to resist aggressive impulses that result in serious assaultive acts of destruction of property where the degree of aggressiveness is grossly out of proportion to any precipitating psychosocial stressors and not better accounted for by another mental disorder[3]. A large epidemiological study of the general population, the National Comorbidity Survey found that IED has a lifetime prevalence of 5.4% in the United States; nearly 40% of those surveyed met diagnostic criteria for IED by age 10 years and the average age of onset for IED was 14 years. Of note, 81% of people in the general population who met diagnostic criteria for IED in this survey also met diagnostic criteria for at least one other Diagnostic and Statistical Manual of Mental Disorders, Fourth Edition psychiatric disorder, most commonly anxiety disorders, impulse control disorders, mood disorders, and substance abuse disorders[4]. "Bullying" is a type of pathological proactive aggression also common in the general population. It has been estimated that close to half of all children are bullied at one point while in the primary or secondary school and at least 10 percent of children are bullied regularly. Bullying is defined as aggressive behaviors that are repeated over time as a means of getting what one wants through coercion or force. These negative, unwanted behaviors are used to establish some sort of perceived superiority or power over another person. Bullying can take many forms including: verbal attacks and name-calling; physical intimidation through hitting, kicking, shoving or spitting; psychological attacks through social exclusion or isolation, spreading lies or false rumors, and/or forcing someone to do things. Bullies can also victimize by using the cell phone or internet to terrorize or humiliate individuals (i.e. "Cyber bullying").

Bullying generally begins in the elementary grades, peaks in middle school, and persists into high school. In some cases, bullying behaviors persist well into adulthood. Bullying behaviors in adults usually have childhood antecedents of bullying, being bullied, or both. Overall, both bullying and being bullied are more common among males. Male bullies are also much more likely than females to use physical intimidation. Female bullies are more likely to use verbal and/ or "relational aggression" (e.g. social exclusion, spreading rumors).

Bullying behaviors pose serious public health hazards for all. Being bullied is associated with increased rates of depression, psychotic symptoms, suicide, self-injurious behaviors, anxiety, and school avoidance. In addition, bullying behavior is associated with adult sociopathy, alcohol and substance abuse, poor academics, and interpersonal and occupational outcomes.

AGGRESSIVE SYMPTOMS IN TS

Aggressive symptoms in people with TS have been described worldwide and appear to be relatively common in clinic populations. Most aggressive behaviors in TS are "reactive" and first manifest in childhood. Aggression can be directed at self, others, and/or objects. While there is some debate about the relationship of aggressive symptoms with the underlying tic diathesis, most studies show that these symptoms rarely occur in TS with tics only. The following section will highlight self-injurious behaviors, explosive outbursts ("rage attacks"), and bullying since these particular aggressive symptoms are the most commonly experienced by people with TS.

SELF-INJURIOUS BEHAVIORS IN TS

Self-injurious behaviors (SIB) are deliberate, non-accidental, repetitive infliction of self-harm without suicidal intent. Examples of SIB include: skin and scab picking, nail biting, hair pulling, scratching, punching or pinching oneself, head or fist banging, teeth grinding and self-biting. SIB occurs in approximately 4% of the general psychiatric population and is most frequently associated with borderline personality disorder, eating disorders, and psychoactive substance abuse. For people with these problems, SIB functions as a way to relieve tension, control affect, or serve as penance for a perceived wrong doing. SIB is also common in certain neurodevelopmental disorders such as Lesch-Nyhan syndrome, Prader-Wili syndrome or autism where such symptoms are associated with pervasive neurological dysfunction.

SIB has been reported more frequently in people with TS than in the general population. The large international study of TS by Freeman and colleagues (2000), reported SIB in 14% of all patients with TS, with higher SIB rates associated with increasing number of comorbid psychiatric disorders, particularly attention deficit hyperactivity disorder (ADHD) and Obsessive Compulsive Disorder (OCD)[1].

SIB has also been correlated with severity of tic symptoms and with high levels of Obsessionality[5]. Mild/moderate cases of SIB may be related to obsessive compulsive symptoms whereas severe SIB cases seem more related to impulsivity alone[6]. Mild/moderate SIB also often appears more tic—or compulsion-like in character and context, whereas severe SIB is more usually accompanied by prominent mood dysregulation and broader problems with impulse control.

Case #5—Self-Injurious Behaviors

Johnny is a 14 year old boy with TS, ADHD, OCD, and depression. He has recently experienced an overall worsening of tic symptoms, coinciding with starting high school. He has also had a recurrence of compulsive skin and cuticle picking which has become so severe that one of his nail beds became infected. He describes an uncomfortable sensation that makes him feel that he has to pick the skin until it feels "just right." He finds this urge to pick "irresistible" despite the untoward and painful consequences.

CARNEGIE PUBLIC LIBRARY
202 N Animas St
Trinidad, CO 81082-2643
(719) 846-6841

EXPLOSIVE OUTBURSTS IN TS

Explosive outbursts, or "rage attacks" occur in both children and adults with TS and are phenomenologically similar to IED. These dramatic symptoms of reactive aggression include recurrent episodes of severe verbal and/or physical aggression that occur with little to no apparent provocation or are grossly out of proportion to the precipitating stressor. These episodes are experienced as uncontrollable, unwanted, and distressing. Those who suffer from these symptoms usually experience enormous shame, embarrassment, and remorse. For their loved ones, life begins to feel scary and unpredictable, "like walking on egg shells." Usually, the trigger is a relatively minor frustration, such as a last minute change in plans or a parent's negative response (i.e. "No!") to a request. While these explosive outbursts may occur elsewhere, in the overwhelming majority of cases, they occur at home and are directed at one (usually mother) or both parents. Siblings, pets, and/or property are also targets. Toxic, hateful expletives or accusations are screamed, holes punched in walls, heavy furniture overturned or thrown, and physical assault with bodily injury can occur. Persons with explosive outbursts often experience a sense of mounting inner tension just prior to the attack, followed by a feeling of physical relief and exhaustion once the episode has terminated. Although most explosive outbursts are quite intense but relatively brief in duration, in some cases episodes last for quite some time or may recur several times throughout the day.

Preliminary research suggests that there are potentially six factors that influence the character of these explosive outbursts: 1) a "compulsion mediated" component, which refers to whether or not an uncomfortable cognitive and/or sensory urge was experienced prior to a rage attack; 2) a "situation mediated" factor, which refers to whether rage is associated with specific situations or environmental settings and also tends to be associated with anticipatory anxiety and occurrence of episodes outside the home; 3) an "impulse associated" factor that is associated with lack of premeditation and quick response to a given stimulus; 4) a "relational associated" component that describes a reactive state associated with a relationship between the child and another individual; 5) a "lability associated" factor that refers to arousal resolution following the outburst (i.e. whether the child is able to return to normal or remains in a hyper—aroused state); and 6) a "control

CASPHERT PUBLIC LIBRARY
202 H Aun... St
Tu...l, CJ 81032-2613
1A8u-0A8 (21)

associated" factor, which relates to the degree that the child is able to voluntarily suppress rage and/or tics[7].

Tics alone do not appear linked with increased aggressive behaviors, although some studies report an association between overall tic severity and aggressive symptoms. Most research in this area emphasizes the association between explosive outbursts and psychiatric comorbidity[8-9]. ADHD has been consistently linked with aggressive symptoms in children with and without tics. In several studies of children with TS, the presence and severity of ADHD are the main predictors of disruptive behaviors including aggression, with no significant correlation between tic severity and ADHD severity. Nonetheless, the complex interactions and relationships among multiple concurrent psychiatric comorbidities, medications, development, and environment are dynamic and difficult to untangle in many instances. For this reason, the presence of explosive outbursts in a person with TS requires very careful and comprehensive assessment.

Environmental factors such as parenting style, family traits (i.e. high expressed emotion, low cohesiveness, highly controlling), highly conflictual or aggressive marital relationship, psychiatric illness in one or both parents (or siblings), peer acceptance, and school experiences are also important influences on aggressive behaviors in TS. Since TS often has a genetic component, one or both parents (and siblings) may be also wrestling with their own symptoms of anxiety, depression or mood dysregulation, compulsivity, distractibility, and/or impulsivity that further challenge effective parenting. It is also possible that when parents show increased attention and submission to their child's aggressive behaviors, especially on an intermittent basis, these symptoms may be inadvertently reinforced.

Case #6—The Classic Rage Attack

Anthony is an 11 year old boy with TS, ADHD, Oppositional Defiant Disorder, OCD, and non-OCD anxiety. Although he has had temper tantrums in the past, his parents are concerned about a new level of explosive behavior that occurs episodically and seems to come out of the blue. His mother says that without warning, Anthony's anger escalates "from zero to 10." In those rare instances when she can identify a potential trigger, it always seems so grossly disproportionate to his responses. During these episodes, he cannot be reasoned with;

he screams devastatingly hurtful things and even punches holes in the wall. Afterwards, he usually expresses remorse but this doesn't appear to prevent him from having another episode.

BULLYING BEHAVIORS AND TS

Bullying is an important type of aggression that affects many people with TS. In the majority of cases, children with TS are victims or bully-victims (i.e. both a bully and a victim). Having a chronic medical, behavioral, emotional or developmental disability can label an individual as "different" and put him/her at a higher risk for criticism and ostracism by classmates. This kind of peer victimization in patients with TS is correlated with tic symptom severity, loneliness, anxiety, and parent reports of child internalizing symptoms[10]. When ostracism from peers is combined with the higher likelihood of suffering from ADHD, OCD and non-OCD anxiety disorders, depression, certain learning disabilities and medication-related side effects such as weight gain and cognitive dulling, findings of decreased social functioning and impaired peer relations are not surprising. There is also evidence from the internet-based omnibus Tourette Syndrome Impact Survey that children with TS who are bullied are more likely to have rage attacks[11]. It appears that only a minority of children with TS become bullies as well as bully-victims. However, although many children and adults with TS report having experienced bullying at least at some point during their lives, the prevalence and scope of this problem has not been fully ascertained and additional research is urgently required.

Case #7—Peer Victimization in TS

Nancy is a 15 year old female with TS, ADHD, OCD, panic attacks, and recurrent depression. Recently she has begun complaining about a variety of somatic symptoms such as headaches and stomachaches. She refuses to go to school in the morning, insisting that she feels "sick." After much exploration, Nancy finally admits that a group of girls at school have spread terrible rumors about her on the internet and accused her of being "a slut." Nancy fears any encounter with this group of girls. She has tried to solicit support from school staff in the past, but was always told that she was being "too sensitive" and that ignoring bullies would make them go away. Hence, school has become a hostile, unsafe environment for Nancy.

TREATMENT OF AGGRESSIVE SYMPTOMS IN TS

Since the nature of aggressive symptoms in TS varies, there is no single "one size fits all" recommended treatment. Instead, interventions must be tailored to individual circumstances, usually incorporating pharmacological and non-pharmacological interventions.

It is helpful to first qualify and quantify certain aspects of the aggressive symptoms at baseline and then again after treatment, to assess whether a given intervention has been effective in reducing overall aggression severity. Formal rating scales of aggressive symptoms (e.g. the Overt Aggression Scale) have been developed for research purposes. The TS Rage Severity Scale was devised as a relatively quick clinical measure to rate changes in certain parameters of aggressive symptoms over time (see Table #3).

Table 3: TS Rage Severity Scale, Budman & Coffey (2004)

Score	0	1	2	3
Frequency (in past week)	None	1-2	3-7	> 1 per day
Intensity (most severe of past week)	Absent	Mild (i.e. temper tantrum)	Moderate (i.e. property destruction)	Severe (i.e. requires hospitalization)
Duration (most severe of past week)	None	≤ 5 min.	6-15 min.	≥ 16 min.
Total Score:				
Mild: 0-3		Moderate: 4-6		Severe: 7-9

In general, reactive ("impulsive") aggression is treated with medication management, whereas non-reactive ("predatory") aggression responds better to non-pharmacological, behavioral interventions. However, in many cases optimal treatment of aggressive symptoms in TS requires a combination of both medications and behavioral therapies. The selection of a particular medication or medication combination is decided after first identifying the most likely psychiatric or medical condition causing aggressive symptoms.

If a medication adverse effect or drug interaction is suspected, then attempting to withdraw and discontinue the putative offending agent is the best initial approach.

Once possible medication side effects and underlying medical, neurological problems, and/or prominent psycho-social causes have been excluded as primary etiologies, it is essential to identify possible psychiatric comorbidities and determine which ones, alone or in combination, may be generating or sustaining aggressive symptoms. In most cases, comorbid ADHD, OCD, and/or Mood Disorders emerge as the primary focus for treatment, with tic stabilization taking a necessary backseat.

As a rule of thumb, stabilization of mood and anxiety (i.e. depression, mania, mixed states, OCD and non-OCD anxiety) receives first priority. Once mood is stabilized, treatment of other psychiatric conditions is prioritized and is approached systematically. If mood is stable, ADHD can be safely addressed in most cases with relatively little risk of exacerbating tic symptoms and considerable benefit in terms of decreasing aggressive symptoms. Psychostimulants are particularly useful for treatment of aggressive symptoms associated with ADHD, but reports showed diminished efficacy for aggression—related behaviors when comorbid conduct disorder or mental retardation is present. Additionally, recent studies provide evidence for using the α-adrenergic agent, clonidine, either alone or in combination with psychostimulant for treatment of aggression in children with ADHD and tic disorders[12]. In the case of comorbid OCD, many of the same medications used to treat depression and/or anxiety are also used at higher doses to treat OCD, typically (although not always) with little impact on tics. In many instances, improvement of OCD symptoms is associated with an overall improvement in tic symptoms. An overview of different psychopharmacological agents used to treat aggressive symptoms in TS is summarized in Table #4. Most of these agents are used either alone or in combination as indicated.

Table 4: Possible Treatments for Aggression in TS

Possible Medication Treatments for Aggression Dysregualtion in TS	
Atypical Antipsychotics	risperidone, aripiprazole, olanzapine, ziprasidone, quetiapine
SSRIs	fluoxetine, sertraline, fluvoxamine, citalopram, escitalopram, paroxetine
Mood Stabilizers/ Anticonvulsants	lithium, divalproex, lamotrigine, carbamazepine, topiramate
α-adrenergic agents	clonidine, guanfacine
Psychostimulants	methylphenidate derivatives, amphetamine and mixed amphetamine salt preparations
Other	propranolol, mecamylamine

Conventional first generation or "typical" antipsychotics such as haloperidol, fluphenazine, and pimozide have been associated with side effects such as sedation, elevated serum prolactin, tardive dyskinesia and parkinsonian symptoms. Non-conventional second generation or "atypical" antipsychotics have been found to be especially efficient in treatment of aggressive symptoms and may have fewer undesirable side effects. This category includes: risperidone, olanzapine, quetiapine, ziprazidone and aripiprazole. Two of these medications, risperidone and aripiprazole have already demonstrated efficacy in decreasing aggressive symptoms in autisim[13-14]. Small clinical studies in children with TS and aggressive symptoms suggest that risperidone, olanzapine, and aripriprazole are helpful in reducing the frequency and intensity of outbursts and also reduce tics[15-18].

Selective Serotonin Reuptake Inhibitors (SSRIs) such as fluoxetine, fluvoxamine and sertraline have been the most extensively studied for the treatment of impulsive aggression in non-TS patients with borderline personality disorder, major depression, and IED. However, the SSRIs may be helpful for treating aggression in TS. An open label study using the SSRI paroxetine was shown to decrease severity and frequency of rage attacks in children and adults with TS[19]. Unfortunately, a small group of people with TS experience untoward effects from SSRIs such as increased agitation, suicidal ideation and even worsening or new-onset aggression, so cautious selection of patients and careful medication titrations with close supervision are important. Larger, well-controlled clinical trials using SSRIs to target aggressive symptoms in TS are needed.

Mood stabilizers such as lithium or the anticonvulsants carbamazepine, divalproex, and lamogtrogine have shown efficacy in placebo-controlled trials for treating aggressive symptoms in adolescents with explosive outbursts, in children with conduct disorder, and in adult patients with personality disorders[20-23]. A retrospective chart review of 41 TS patients treated with topiramate revealed improvement in both tics and aggressive symptoms[24]. Further studies are warranted to explore potential clinical applications of these medications for treatment of aggressive symptoms in TS.

Non-pharmacologic interventions are important as primary or adjunctive treatment of aggression in TS. While some of these treatments are highly specific, many are potentially synergistic (e.g. marital therapy and parent management training, exercise and collaborative problem solving). A complete description of each treatment is beyond the scope of this chapter; some of the common non-pharmacological options are summarized in Table #5 (see Table #5 below).

Table 5: Non-Medication Treatments for Aggressive Symptoms in TS

Non-Medication Treatments for Aggressive Symptoms in TS		
Psychoeducation	Anger Management Programs	School In-Service on TS
Parent Management Training	(incl. Anger Control Training, ACT)	"TS Ambassador Program"
Family Therapy	Collaborative Problem Solving	Physical Exercise
Marital Therapy	Dialectical Behavioral Therapy Cognitive Behavioral Therapy	Nutrition/Diet/Sleep Hygiene

While a variety of non-pharmacological interventions may be helpful for reducing aggressive symptoms in TS, surprisingly few have been formally studied in this particular population. Anger control training appears effective for mild to moderate aggression symptoms in TS. In a randomized trial assessing the efficacy of ten sessions of individually administered Anger Control Training for adolescents with TS and aggressive symptoms, subjects were assigned to either anger control training or "treatment as usual". Subjects in the anger control training had significantly decreased scores on the Disruptive Behavior Rating Scale when compared with the "treatment as usual group"[25]. Parent training is essential in helping the parent understand and properly deal with their child's condition; this includes self-education and psychosocial treatments. A specific type of parent training developed by Kazdin is Parental Management Training, which emphasizes active parental training in the application of targeted positive reinforcement (i.e. "operant conditioning.") Parents are encouraged to frequently praise prosocial, appropriate behaviors, while also applying predictable and consistent consequences for disruptive behaviors. Parental Management Training uncovers parent-child interactions that inadvertently reinforce disruptive behaviors, and instead shifts parental focus towards building the child's adaptive skills. It has demonstrated efficacy as a parental therapy for children with autistic spectrum disorders, conduct disorder, oppositional defiant disorder, and ADHD, but there has been little research on children with TS specifically[26]. Collaborative Problem Solving is another important cognitive behavioral intervention that assumes oppositional defiant or aggressive behaviors stem largely from a skills deficit and therefore engages both parent and child in a cooperative dialogue about how to develop particular strategies for addressing problem behaviors, such as tolerating frustration, being flexible, and avoiding emotional overreaction[27].

CONCLUSION

As is the case with many other medical and psychiatric illnesses, affected individuals with TS and their families learn to cope with most challenges and symptoms. Yet, when present, aggressive symptoms are highly likely to have a negative impact on overall disease burden and can lead to residential placements, severe family conflicts, marital estrangement and divorce, "burn-out" and social isolation. For these reasons, identifying and treating such symptoms when present are of paramount importance. As our understanding of the bio-psycho-social underpinnings of aggression in TS expands, improved treatment outcomes can be expected.

References

1. Freeman, R., Fast, D., Burd, L., (2000) An international perspective on Tourette Syndrome: Selected findings from 3500 cases in 22 countries. *Dev Med Child Neurol* **42**, 436-447.

2. Dooley, J., Brna, P. & Gordon, K. (1999) Parent perceptions of symptom severity in Tourette's syndrome. *Arch Dev Child* **81**, 440-441.

3. American Psychiatric Association. (2000) *Diagnostic and Statistical Manual of Mental Disorders, Fourth edition Text revision.* American Psychiatric Association, Washington, D.C.

4. Kessler, R.C., Coccaro, E.F., Fava, M., Jaegar, S., Jin, R. & Walters, E. (2006) **The Prevalence and Correlates of *DSM-IV* Intermittent Explosive Disorder in the National Comorbidity Survey Replication.** *Arch Gen Psychiatry* **63**, 669- 678.

5. Robertson, M., Trimble, M. & Lees, A. (1989) Self-injurious behavior and the Gilles de la Tourette syndrome: a clinical study and review of the literature. *Psychol Med* **19**, 611-625.

6. Mathews, C.A., Waller, J., Glidden, D.V., Lowe, T.L., Herrera, L.D., Budman, C.L., Erenberg, G., Naarden, A., Bruun, R.D., Freimer, N.B. & Reus, V.I. (2004) Self injurious behavior in Tourette syndrome: correlates with impulsivity and impulse control. *J Neurol Neurosurg Psychiatry* **75**, 1149- 1155.

7. Budman, C.L., Rockmore, L., Stokes, J., & Sossin, M. (2003) Clinical phenomenology of episodic rage in children with Tourette Syndrome. *J Psychosom Res* **55**, 59-65.

8. Budman, C.L., Bruun, R.D., Park, K.S., Lesser, M. & Olson, M. (2000) Explosive outbursts in children with Tourette's disorder. *J Am Acad Child Adolesc Psychiatry* **39(10)**, 1270- 1275.

9. Stephens, R. & Sandor, P. (1999) Aggressive behavior in children with Tourette syndrome and comorbid attention- deficit hyperactivity disorder and obsessive- compulsive disorder. *Can J Psychiatry* **44**, 1036- 1042.

10. Storch, W., Murphy, T., Chase, R., Keeley, M., Jann, K., Murray, M., Geffken, G.R. (2007) Peer victimization in youth with Tourette's syndrome and chronic tic disorder: Relations with tic severity and internalizing symptoms. *J Psychopathol Behav Assess* **29**, 211-219.

11. Conelea, C., Woods, D.W., Zinner, S.H., Budman, C.L., Murphy, T., Scahill, L.D., Compton, S.N., & Walkup, J. (2011) Exploring the impact of Tourette syndrome on youth: Results from the Tourette syndrome impact survey. *J Child Psychiatry Human Dev* **42(2),** 219-242.

12. Budman, C.L. (2006) Treatment of aggression in Tourette Syndrome. *Adv Neurol* **99,** 222- 226.

13. Shea, S., Turgay, A., Carroll, A., Schultz, M. Orlik, H., Smith, I. & Dunbar, F. (2004) Risperidone in the treatment of disruptive behavioral symptoms in children with autistic and other pervasive developmental disorders. *Pediatrics* **114(4),** e634-641.

14. Owen, R., Sikich, L., Marcus, R.N., Corey-Lisle, P., Manos, G., McQuade,R.D.,Carson,W.H.&Findling,R.L.(2009)Aripiprazole in the treatment of irritability in children and adolescents with autistic disorder. *Pediatrics* **124(6),** 1533- 1540.

15. Sandor, P. & Stephens, R. (2000) Risperidone treatment of aggressive behavior in children with Tourette's syndrome. *J Clin Psychopharmacol* **20,** 710-712.

16. Stephens, R.J., Basse, C. & Sandor, P. (2004) Olanzapine in the treatment of aggression and tics in children with Tourette's syndrome--a pilot study. *J Child Adolesc Psychopharmacol.* **14(2),** 255-266.

17. Scahill, L., Leckman, J.F., Schultz, R.T., Katsovich, L. & Peterson, B.S. (2003) A placebo- controlled trial of risperidone in Tourette syndrome. *Neurology* **60,** 1130-1135.

18. Budman, C.L., Coffey, B.J., Shechter, R., Schrock, M., Wieland, N., Spirgel, A. & Simon, E. (2008) Aripiprazole in children and adolescents with Tourette disorder with and without explosive outbursts. *J Child Adolesc Psychopharmacol* **18(5),** 509-515.

19. Bruun, R.D. & Budman, C.L. (1998) Paroxetine treatment of episodic rages associated with Tourette disorder. *J Clin Psychiatry* **59(11),** 581-584.

20. Campbell, M., Adams, P., Small, A.M., Kafantaris, V., Silva, R.R., Shell, J., Perry, R. & Overall, J.E. (1995) Lithium in hospitalized aggressive children with conduct disorder: a double-blind and placebo=controlled study. *J Am Acad Child Adolesc Psychiatry* **34,** 445-453.

21. Donovan, S., Stewart, J., Nunes, E., Quitkin, F.M., Parides, M., Daniel, W., Susser, E. & Klein, D.F. (2000) Divalproex treatment for youth with explosive temper and mood lability: a double-blind, placebo-controlled crossover design. *Am J Psychiatry* **157,** 818-820.

22. Lewin, J. & Sumners, D. (1992) Successful treatment of episodic dyscontrol with carbamazepine. *Br J Psychiatry* **161,** 261-262.

23. Malone, R., Delaney, M., Luebbert, J.F., Cater, J. & Campbell, M. (2000) A double-blind placebo-controlled study of lithium in hospitalized aggressive children and adolescents with conduct disorder. *Arch Gen Psychiatry* **57,** 649-654.

24. Kuo, S.H. & Jimenez-Shahed, J. (2010) Topiramate in treatment of Tourette syndrome. *Clin Neuropharmacol.* **33(1),** 32- 34.

25. Sukhodolsky, D.G., Vitulano, L.A., Carroll, D.H., McGuire, J., Leckman, J.F. & Scahill, L. (2009) Randomized trial of anger control training for adolescents with Tourette's Syndrome and disruptive behavior. *J Am Acad Child Adolesc Psychiatry* **48(4),** 413- 421.

26. Sukhodolsky, D.G. (2006) [Review of the book *Parent management training: Treatment for oppositional, aggressive, and antisocial behavior in children and adolescents,* by AE Kazdin]. *J Am Acad Child Adolesc Psychiatry* **45(2),** 256-257.

27. Greene, R.W., Ablon, J.S. & Goring, J.C. (2003) A transactional model of oppositional behavior: Underpinnings of the Collaborate Problem Solving approach. *J Psychosom Res* **55(1),** 67- 75.

CHAPTER 5

HOW COMMON IS TOURETTE SYNDROME IN CHILDREN?

Lawrence Scahill, M.S.N., Ph.D.

INTRODUCTION

The first cases of TS were described over 100 years ago. The patients were all adults and all had severe tics. The prevailing view for several decades that followed presumed that TS was an extraordinarily rare condition and uniformly severe. Things have changed and this is no longer the prevailing view. The contemporary view, based on all available evidence, is that the tics of TS range from mild to severe. This change in viewpoint has a major impact on the answer to the question posed in the title of this article. The purpose of this chapter is to provide up to date answers for this question.

PREVALENCE

The term *prevalence* is used to describe how common a condition is in the population. It is a simple fraction comprised of the number of cases with a given condition divided by the number of people in the population of interest. For example, the number of children with TS in a specific geographical area divided by all children living in that region would be a statement of prevalence. In common conditions such as Attention Deficit Hyperactivity Disorder (ADHD), prevalence is expressed as cases per 100. In less commonly occurring conditions, such as TS, prevalence is often expressed as cases per 1000 or 10,000.

$$\text{Prevalence} = \frac{\text{number of cases}}{\text{population of interest}}$$

Because TS is not usually evident in children under the age of 5 years, studies of prevalence are often focused on children between the ages of 6 and 17 years—rather than all children. The formula above illustrates that prevalence is all about counting cases. Although the definition of prevalence is relatively simple, counting cases of TS can be complicated. There is no blood test, X-ray, brain scan or any diagnostic laboratory test for TS. The diagnosis is made by obtaining a careful history of motor and phonic tics as well as observation during the assessment.

PREVALENCE OF TICS AND TIC DISORDERS IN CHILDHOOD

The prevalence of TS is not just an intellectual curiosity. Disorders such as TS that begin in childhood can affect a child's short—and long-term adjustment in interpersonal, educational and occupational domains. Reliable estimates on the prevalence of TS could inform planning for medical, psychological and educational services. Among the many issues to be resolved in obtaining a trustworthy prevalence estimate of TS is the definition. The definition is likely to consider the number and types of tics as well as the duration of the tics. For example, it has been shown that isolated and temporary tics are common in school-age children with estimates ranging from 10% to 20%. These isolated tics that do not endure over time do not constitute a disorder. Children with mild sporadic tics are rarely bothered by the tics, which often go unnoticed by others.

The current official listing of tic disorders (the Diagnostic and Statistical Manual of Mental Disorders, Fourth Edition) defines four types that are relevant to the current discussion. Transient Tic Disorder consists of motor tics, vocal tics or both lasting at least two weeks, but less than one year. Chronic Tic Disorder is defined by the presence of motor or vocal tics (but not both) lasting for more than a year. Tourette's disorder (also known as Tourette syndrome) includes multiple motor tics and at least one vocal tic lasting for a more than a year (see Chapter 2).

Table 1: Current Definition Of Tic Disorders		
Tic Disorder Type	**Tic Type**	**Duration**
Transient	Motor, phonic or both	At least 2 weeks, less than one year
Chronic Motor	Motor	Greater than one year
Chronic Vocal	Vocal	Greater than one year
Tourette syndrome	Multiple motor and at least one vocal	Greater than one year

After settling on the definition of tic disorders, the next important step is selecting a sample to be surveyed. First and foremost, the survey should include a sample from the community. This is essential because not all children with TS or related tic disorders make their way to a clinic. Indeed, every community survey conducted over the past 20 years has counted cases of TS that had not been previously diagnosed. This repeated observation underscores the notion that children referred for treatment may not be representative of all children with TS. Thus, to obtain a trustworthy estimate of prevalence, it is necessary to go beyond cases from clinical settings and evaluate community samples.

The next research challenge is the method of assessment. Some studies rely on pencil and paper checklists from parents, teachers or both. These approaches are attractive because they are relatively inexpensive. However, the diagnosis may not be accurate. Some cases of TS may be missed and some children who do not have TS may be misclassified. A better approach is to ask detailed questions of the parent to learn about the onset and course of tics. This takes more time and costs more than gathering pencil and paper checklists, but is more accurate. In addition to direct interviews with a parent, some studies include face-to-face examination and observation of the child. This is probably the most accurate diagnostic approach, but also the most expensive.

Over the past decade, ten community surveys in children focusing on the prevalence of TS have been conducted. The sample sizes ranged from 475 to 9,000 children. Although most studies applied diagnostic definitions that are consistent with those listed in Table 1, the estimates of prevalence for TS showed a wide range (from 3 to 38 per 1,000 children). These differences have to do with sample size, diagnostic assessment (simple checklists versus detailed interviews), and the rate of participation in the study (some studies had very low participation rate). Small samples and low participation rate in the survey are likely to produce unreliable estimates because the study sample may not be a fair representation of all children in the community.

To arrive at a best estimate for the prevalence of TS in children, it seems fair to disregard four studies with less than 1000 children, one study with a very low participation rate, and one other study that used a somewhat different definition of TS. The four remaining studies provide an estimate of about 6 per 1,000 children. Table 2 presents the predicted number of cases based on various prevalence estimates and an estimated 50 million school-age children in the United States.

Table 2: Actual Number of TS Cases In School-Age Children Based On A Range Of Prevalence Estimates		
Prevalence Estimate Per 1,000 Children	US Population of School-age Children	Number of TS Cases Nationwide
3		150,000
6	50,000,000	300,000
8		400,000
10		500,000

NUMBER OF CHILDREN SEEKING TREATMENT FOR TS

The Centers for Disease Control and Prevention (CDC) conducted a nationwide survey of households in 2007-08. Using random digit dialing, the survey included 64,000 households with at least one child between the age of 6 and 17 years. The survey asked parents many questions about health and disease including the presence of TS. For example, parents were asked: "Has a doctor or other health care provider ever told you that your child has Tourette syndrome?" This study resulted in an estimated 3 cases per 1,000—exactly half of our best estimate of 6 per 1,000. As noted above, children who make it to clinic are unlikely to be all cases—some cases go undetected. Most cases were described as mild. Common coexisting problems included ADHD, disruptive behavioral problems and anxiety. One of the remarkable findings from the CDC survey is that the rate of diagnosis was dramatically lower in minority populations (1.5 per 1,000 for Hispanics and 1.6 per 1,000 for African-Americans), compared to white children (3.9 per 1,000). The reasons for this difference are not entirely clear, but may be due to problems of access to care for minority populations.

CONCLUSION

Tics are common in childhood. In many children, tics are isolated and temporary. The best estimate for the prevalence of TS in school-age children is 6 per 1,000 (about 300,000 cases nationwide). Most cases are mild and the tics of TS often improve with age. Nonetheless, children with TS, even those with mild conditions, have a higher likelihood of other problems such as ADHD, disruptive behavior and anxiety. Children with TS alone, regardless of severity, appear to have only slightly greater risk for disability than children in the general population. Therefore, diagnosis and treatment require identification of the most pressing problem rather than focus only on the tics. Data from National Survey of Children's Health by the CDC indicate that a substantial number of children with TS are missed, suggesting that improved recognition is needed. The problem of missing cases appears to be especially acute in minority populations.

References

1. American Psychiatric Association. (2000) Diagnostic and statistical manual of mental disorders. 4th ed. rev. (DSM-IV-R). American Psychiatric Association Press, Washington, D.C.
2. Centers for Disease Control and Prevention (CDC). (2009) Prevalence of diagnosed Tourette syndrome in persons aged 6-17 years – United States, 2007. *MMWR Morb Mort Wkly Rep* **58(21),** 581-585.
3. Hirtz, D., Thurman, D.J., Gwinn-Hardy, K., Mohamed, M., Chaudhuri, A.R. & Zalutsky, R. (2007) How common are the "common" neurologic disorders? *Neurology* **68(5),** 326-337.
4. Robertson, M.M. (2008) The prevalence and epidemiology of Gilles de la Tourette syndrome. *J Psychosomatic Res* **65(5),** 461-486.
5. Scahill, L., Sukhodolsky, D.G., Williams, S.K. & Leckman, J.F. (2005) Public health significance of tic disorders in children and adolescents. *Adv Neurol* **96,** 240-248.
6. Snider, L.A., Seligman, L.D. & Ketchen, B.R. (2002) Tics and problem behaviors in schoolchildren: Prevalence, characterization, and associations. *Pediatrics* **110(2),** 331-336.

CHAPTER 6

THE CAUSES OF TS AND CHANGES THAT OCCUR IN THE BRAIN

Jonathan W. Mink, M.D., Ph.D.

INTRODUCTION

TS is defined by the presence of tics: discrete, stereotyped, repetitive involuntary movements. However, as described in Chapters 2 and 3, many individuals with TS also have other symptoms including inattention, impulsivity, anxiety, obsessive thinking, and compulsive behaviors. Over the past 40-50 years, it has become apparent that the basis for these symptoms lies in altered function of certain brain regions. However, exact mechanisms of this altered function and the specific brain regions involved remain the focus of active research. TS is not caused by damage to a particular part of the brain such as one might see after a stroke. It is also not caused by absence of certain brain regions. Instead, TS is likely to be caused by dysfunction of brain circuits that normally work together to regulate the flow of movements, thoughts, and behavior.

How do we know what brain mechanisms are involved in TS? Historically, much of our knowledge about brain mechanisms in neurologic disorders came from the study of brains from individuals who died with those disorders. However, TS is not associated with any obvious brain injury, degeneration, or malformation, so classic neuropathology methods revealed little about brain mechanisms in TS. Initial thoughts about brain mechanisms in TS came from studies in people with other kinds of movement disorders such as Parkinson disease and Huntington disease. While TS is quite different from those degenerative disorders, their study has led to the understanding of how brain dysfunction can lead to involuntary movements. With the advent of modern neuroimaging, where the structure and function of the human brain can be studied non-invasively in living people, important clues began to emerge. More modern methods in anatomy and chemistry have provided new insights based on the post-mortem study of brains from people with TS. Finally, the development of better animal models have allowed neuroscientists to develop and test more specific hypotheses about brain circuits in TS.

What and where are these brain circuits? The key brain mechanisms involved in TS are thought to be the basal ganglia and the frontal lobes of the cerebral cortex[1]. The basal ganglia are an interconnected group of structures that lie deep in the brain (See Figure 1 below). They are involved in the control of movement and other behaviors by regulating the activity of the frontal lobes and some circuits in the midbrain. The functions of the frontal lobes are complex and many; but a unifying concept is that frontal lobes plan and executes movements, thoughts, and complex behaviors. The basal ganglia appear to act as a "brake" that can be applied to prevent certain movements and behaviors when they are unwanted. At other times, the brake is removed to facilitate those movements and behaviors. Precise regulation of actions is accomplished through a complex interaction between the frontal lobes and the basal ganglia to execute wanted actions and prevent unwanted actions[2,3].

ANATOMIC NEUROIMAGING

Magnetic Resonance Imaging (MRI) has allowed research to examine the structure of the brain non-invasively in living human beings. The high resolution of MRI and the ability to measure brain structures has provided some insights into structural brain differences in TS. The literature on anatomic neuroimaging findings in TS has been somewhat contradictory[1]. This stems in part from the small number of subjects in many of the studies. The anatomic differences between TS brains and non-TS brains are slight and the normal variation of brain size among individuals is such that larger studies are required to provide confidence in the findings. Another source of differences is that some studies include both adults and children. Because most people with TS have improvement or resolution of their symptoms in adulthood, it seems that brain development plays an important role. Thus, it is important to take developmental differences into account in these studies.

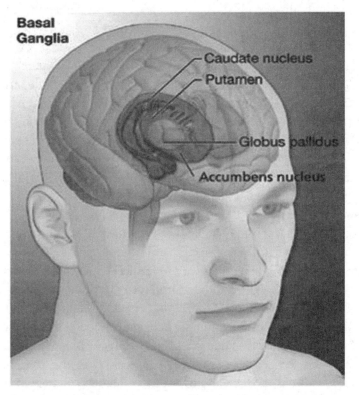

Figure 1. Basal Ganglia: The basal ganglia is a collection of brain structures, located deep within the brain, that are connected via neurons to each other and to other areas of the brain (such as the foremost region called the frontal cortex). These structures normally function in a coordinated manner to control movements. Alterations in one or more structures of the basal ganglia are thought to underlie abnormal movements in various neurological disorders, including the generation of tics in Tourette syndrome.

Early anatomic MRI studies reported conflicting findings about the size of the basal ganglia and other parts of the central nervous system[1]. More recently, larger studies have provided some convergence of findings across studies. Subjects with TS tend to have a smaller size of the caudate nucleus than do normal control subjects[4]. The caudate nucleus is a large "input" structure of the basal ganglia that receives information from the cerebral cortex and processes it in the context of other information. There is also evidence that the sensory and motor parts of the cerebral cortex are thinner in individuals with TS. Individuals with more severe tics appear to have more thinning than do those with mild tics. These findings suggest that differences in the development of interconnected portions of the basal ganglia and cerebral cortex are predisposed to the development of TS. There is also evidence that changes in these and related brain structures may help modulate the severity of symptoms. These are important insights. However, relationships between the size and function of brain parts are complex. A smaller size does not necessarily mean poorer function and a larger size does not mean better function. However, consistent size differences in specific brain regions do suggest that those brain regions are important to understanding the neurobiology of TS.

Another type of anatomic imaging uses a technique called Diffusion Tensor Imaging (DTI). DTI measures directional diffusion of water in the brain. Water diffuses more readily along pathways than across pathways. Thus, DTI can measure properties of pathways that connect one part of the brain with another. Similar to the studies of brain region size, DTI studies have shown conflicting results. Changes in both motor and non-motor parts of the brain have been described [5]. However, there appears to be a consensus that TS subjects have changes in the corpus callosum, the large set of pathways that connect the two cerebral hemispheres. It is less clear how these changes relate to function. However, just as with brain size changes, these findings suggest that understanding differences in the connections between the two sides of the brain may provide important clues about the neurobiology of TS.

FUNCTIONAL IMAGING

Functional imaging typically involves the use of MRI or Positron Emission Tomography to investigate brain function by measuring blood flow patterns (which correlates with brain activity), metabolism, or neurotransmitter systems in living human beings. This is usually done non-invasively or with an injection of short-lasting radioactive tracers. Many functional imaging studies have been performed in TS individuals, but like the anatomic chemical imaging studies, often they have involved very small numbers of subjects. Nevertheless, some common themes have emerged from these studies with most differences between TS subjects and control subjects being found in the basal ganglia, frontal lobes, or the thalamus. The thalamus connects the basal ganglia output with the frontal lobes. Functional imaging studies can be divided into several types of studies based on the technique and the scientific question.

Brain Activity Related to Tics

Perhaps the most obvious question one would like to answer is "what parts of the brain cause tics." This question is harder to answer than one might expect. Three factors contribute to this difficulty. First, precise and accurate imaging requires that the head does not move during imaging. Since most tics involve the upper body, head movement is common. Second, if brain regions change activity in relation to tics it may be difficult to tell whether the change of brain activity caused the tics or if the tics caused the change of brain activity. Even in studies where spontaneously occurring tics were compared to mimicking tics (where the subject makes voluntary movements that are similar to the tics) it is difficult to eliminate confounding factors. One clever approach to solving this problem has involved having TS subjects actively suppress their tics. Tic suppression was associated with activity changes in the basal ganglia and related areas of the frontal lobes[6].

Brain Activity Differences in TS Not Related to Tics

To circumvent some confounds associated with studying brain activity during tics, some scientists have studied patterns of brain activity when people with TS are at rest but not ticcing. Using functional MRI, changes in brain activity as reflected in changes in blood flow can be compared across multiple areas of the brain. Some areas appear to change activity in correlation with other areas. Using a method known as "functional connectivity MRI", scientists can look for correlated networks of brain regions and determine whether they differ in TS or not. It appears that some of these networks in cerebral cortex are functionally immature in subjects with TS compared to control subjects at the same age[7]. Another approach has been to study the activity of brain regions while subjects perform a cognitive or motor task and ask whether the brain activity in individuals with TS is different from brain activity in individuals without TS. Several studies have shown slight differences between TS subjects and control subjects, but these have been small studies and it is difficult to draw conclusions[8].

Neurochemical Studies

PET and other methods have been used to study specific chemical neurotransmitters in the brain. Most studies have focused on dopamine and serotonin because these transmitters are targeted by most pharmacologic treatments for tics and related symptoms. Most studies have involved small numbers of subjects and findings have differed substantially across studies. Nevertheless, several studies have provided evidence for increased activity in the dopamine system that modulates the basal ganglia and frontal lobes[1,8]. It is possible that differences across studies reflect differences in symptom type and severity in the individuals who were studied, but this is not known for certain.

NEUROPATHOLOGY

Historically, much has been learned about what brain areas are involved in specific disorders by examining brain tissue under a microscope. However, several factors have complicated this type of study in TS. TS is not fatal, so people with TS die from other causes. In many of those causes, the brain is affected directly or indirectly so that pathologic changes in the brain are likely to be related to factors other than TS. It is also difficult in many cases to be certain whether the diagnosis of TS during life was accurate. Older studies had suggested changes in a variety of neurotransmitter systems in the basal ganglia. Other studies have shown abnormalities in dopamine markers in the cerebral cortex. However, the findings are difficult to interpret because of small sample size and the limitations noted above. More recent studies have taken advantage of more careful determination of diagnosis during life and of more modern neuroanatomical and neurochemical techniques. The most striking and consistent abnormalities have been found in the basal ganglia. Two small populations of neurons in the basal ganglia are decreased in TS[9]. These are inhibitory neurons that stain positive for parvalbumin and neurons that use the neurotransmitter acetylcholine. They play an important role in regulating the activity of large numbers of other types of basal ganglia neurons. It appears that these neurons are important for maintaining the normal braking mechanisms of the basal ganglia. When these neurons are diminished, the brake is more likely to be "off" in an unwanted manner.

ANIMAL MODELS

In the study of many neurological and psychiatric disorders, the development of animal models has led to substantial advances in knowledge. Unfortunately, few good animal models of TS exist. One approach has been to try to develop models in which the animals have abnormal movements or other behaviors. Some putative TS animal models have been developed in rodents, but rodent behavior is sufficiently different from human behavior that it is difficult to know to what degree these models are valid. Another approach has been to take genetic mutations that have been described in people with TS and to develop mouse models that incorporate those mutations. This has the potential to yield useful knowledge about the neurobiology of TS, but these models are just being developed and tested now. One especially promising model has been developed recently in monkeys[10]. This model is based on the injection of a chemical called bicuculline into the basal ganglia. Bicuculline essentially removes the basal ganglia "brake" and may produce a functional equivalent of removing the parvalbumin neurons that were discussed in the previous section. Monkeys injected with bicuculline developed repetitive involuntary movements that bore a striking similarity to human tics. Monkey models of other movement disorders have been critically important in developing a better understanding of the disorders and for testing new treatments. It is too early to know if the monkey model of tics will bear fruit, but it is the best model yet developed.

CONCLUSION

Substantial advances have been made toward understanding the brain mechanisms of TS. These advances have involved a variety of complementary approaches to studying the brain, with modern neuroimaging and neuropathology playing a major role. While the specific mechanisms responsible for TS have not been revealed, there is a convergence of findings that point to altered function of neural circuits that include the basal ganglia and connected areas of the frontal lobes of the cerebral cortex. These findings suggest that the inability to inhibit unwanted movements and behaviors is a likely mechanism. The most effective currently available treatments appear to target these parts of the brain. This is true of pharmacologic treatments (Chapter 9), neurosurgical treatments (Chapter 12), and behavioral treatments (Chapter 11). Although it is likely that there are several different causes of TS, it is also likely that the difference causes result in dysfunction of the basal ganglia and related areas of the cerebral cortex and that future therapies will likely target these parts of the brain as well.

References

1. Albin, R.L. & Mink, J.W. (2006) Recent advances in Tourette syndrome research. *Trends Neurosci* **29,** 175-182.
2. Mink, J. (2003) The basal ganglia and involuntary movements: Impaired inhibition of competing motor patterns. *Arch Neurol* **60,** 1365-1368.
3. Mink, J.W. (1996) The basal ganglia: Focused selection and inhibition of competing motor programs. *Prog Neurobiol* **50,** 381-425.
4. Plessen, K.J., Bansal, R. & Peterson, B.S. (2009) Imaging evidence for anatomical disturbances and neuroplastic compensation in persons with Tourette syndrome. *J Psychosom Res* **67,** 559-573.
5. Neuner, I., Kupriyanova, Y., Stocker, T., Huang, R., Posnansky, O., Schneider, F., Tittgemeyer, M. & Shah, N.J. (2010) White-matter abnormalities in Tourette syndrome extend beyond motor pathways. *Neuroimage* **51,** 1184-1193.
6. Peterson, B.S., Skudlarski, P., Anderson, A.W., Zhang, H., Gatenby, J.C., Lacadie, C.M., Leckman, J.F. & Gore, J.C. (1998) A functional magnetic resonance imaging study of tic suppression in Tourette syndrome. *Arch Gen Psychiatry* **55,** 326-333.
7. Church, J.A., Fair, D.A., Dosenbach, N.U., Cohen, A.L., Miezin, F.M., Peterson, S.E. & Schlagger, B.L. (2009) Control networks in paediatric Tourette syndrome show immature and anomalous patterns of functional connectivity. *Brain* **132,** 225-238.
8. Rickards, H. (2009) Functional neuroimaging in Tourette syndrome. *J Psychosom Res* **67,** 575-584.
9. Kataoka, Y., Kalanithi, P.S., Grantz, H. (2010) Decreased number of parvalbumin and cholinergic interneurons in the striatum of individuals with Tourette syndrome. *J Comp Neurol* **518,** 277-291.
10. McCairn, K.W., Bronfeld, M., Belelovsky, K. & Bar-Gad, I. (2009) The neurophysiological correlates of motor tics following focal striatal disinhibition. *Brain* **132,** 2125-2138.

CHAPTER 7

INHERITANCE, GENES, AND TS

Jeremiah M. Scharf, M.D., Ph.D. and Carol A. Mathews, M.D.

INTRODUCTION

Since the early 1980s, TS researchers have observed that many individuals with the disorder have at least one other family member with TS or a related tic disorder. This tendency for TS to be passed down from one generation to another (known as "inheritance") indicates that genetic factors (which scientists classify into functional units called "genes") play a significant role in determining whether a person will develop TS or not. At the same time, research over the past thirty years has also shown that the inheritance of TS is complex, and that genes alone are probably not the only cause. This chapter aims to describe what is currently known about the genetics of TS and how genetic and non-genetic factors are thought to contribute to TS and related conditions.

WHY IS THE STUDY OF TS GENETICS IMPORTANT?

The search for "TS genes" is a crucial way for researchers to identify the underlying cause of an inherited condition like TS. Genes are stretches of DNA (Deoxyribonucleic Acid) inside every cell of the human body and are thought to serve as a blueprint that encodes and directs the basic biological processes of cells and tissues (See Figure 1 below). When the DNA blueprint of a gene does not work correctly (due to a change in the DNA sequence, known as a "mutation"), the altered gene triggers changes in the function of the body's cells and tissues that result in disease (see Figure 2 below). Therefore, identification of "TS genes" would provide important insight into the fundamental mechanisms inside nerve cells that cause TS. Better knowledge of these mechanisms could lead to improved diagnosis and/or new approaches to treatment.

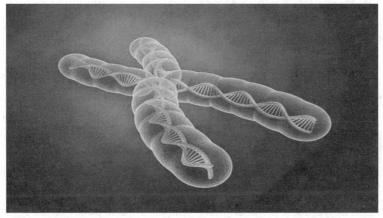

Figure 1. Chromosome/DNA Helix: Every cell in the body, including neurons, contains 23 pairs of chromosomes. Each chromosome is made up of DNA which when condensed and viewed using sophisticated laboratory equipment, appears like the structure above. Individual DNA molecules, when unpacked from the dense chromosome, consist of two spiraling strands known as a double helix.

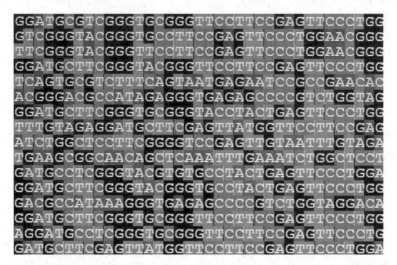

Figure 2. DNA Sequence: Close examination of the composition of DNA shows that it is made up of a sequence of different molecules (called bases). These

molecules have been assigned various letters: A, G, T or C. It is a specific sequence of letters that is referred to as a gene. There are thousands of genes (sequences of letters) in a cell and each gene carries a different piece of information necessary to instruct the cell on how it should function. In Tourette syndrome, there is some evidence that specific genes have been altered (mutated), but we do not yet know the vast majority of genes that are altered or how these alterations cause TS.

STUDIES OF TS INHERITANCE

Before scientists can look for specific genes that predispose individuals to developing TS, the first step is to ask "how genetic" it is. Very few disorders are 100% genetic, and TS is no exception. Therefore, scientists have studied the inheritance patterns or heritability (the percent of TS cases that are caused by genetic factors) of TS by looking at how often TS recurs in families and the specific ways in which TS is passed down through different generations.

TWIN STUDIES

Twin studies are an excellent way to determine whether genes, non-genetic factors (typically called "environmental factors"), or a combination of the two are important in causing a condition like TS. For example, in a condition that is 100% genetic, identical twins (who share 100% of their DNA in common) would both have the condition 100% of the time, whereas non-identical twins, who share only 50% of their DNA, would both have the condition only 50% of the time or less. If inherited conditions like TS are less than 100% genetic, the percent of identical and non-identical twins both having TS would decrease with decreasing genetic contributions. That is; when a condition is "less genetic" and "more environmental", the rate of twins having TS is similar for identical and non-identical twins. These differences allow researchers to estimate the relative contributions of genes and environmental factors to the development of a particular inherited condition.

There are only a few twin studies available for TS, but these studies indicate that TS is strongly genetic and highly heritable[1]. For example, early studies in small numbers of families have shown that when one identical twin had TS, the second twin in the pair also had TS about 55% to 65% of the time. In contrast, in the same studies, non-identical twin pairs both had TS only 8% of the time. This large increase in shared TS between identical twins compared to non-identical twins suggests that genetic factors in general play a major role in determining if someone has TS (though it does not indicate what those specific genetic factors are). However, the fact that the rate of shared TS in identical twins is much less than 100% shows that non-genetic factors are also important (see "Non-genetic contributions" section below). More recent research in very large samples of identical and non-identical twins taken from twin registries who were selected from the general population show similar findings to the original twin studies, with higher rates of both TS and tics in identical twins compared to non-identical twins[2-3]. These findings taken from the general population provide additional support to the hypothesis that both genetic and non-genetic factors play a role in causing TS.

Interestingly, the twin studies also raise the possibility that TS itself may not be the most heritable or "genetic" form of tic disorder, but that the broader category of any chronic tic disorder (TS, chronic motor tics only or chronic vocal tics only) might be more heritable than TS alone. Specifically, these studies showed that when one identical twin had *either* TS *or* chronic motor or vocal tics (CT), the rate of chronic tics (including TS) in the co-twin was 77-94% (compared to only 55-65% when considering only full-blown TS in the co-twin). This increase of shared chronic tics compared to the rate of shared TS only between co-twins argues that researchers should consider both TS and CT together when looking for TS genes in families. At the same time, these results also imply that non-genetic, "environmental" factors may be important in determining whether a particular person who has a genetic susceptibility to tics will develop TS or whether they will develop chronic motor tics alone or chronic vocal tics alone.

FAMILY STUDIES

Scientists also try to determine "how genetic" a condition like TS may be by studying how often TS is present in family members of a TS-affected individual. Family studies have shown that first-degree relatives (parents, children and siblings) of a person with TS have approximately a 5-15% chance of also having TS[4]. When this rate is compared to the occurrence of TS in the general population (approximately 0.5-1% (see Chapter 5)), this leads to the calculation that a first-degree relative has a 10 to 30-fold increased risk of developing TS compared to the risk of TS in the general population (5-15% divided by 0.5-1%). It is important to realize, however, that this increase in TS risk for close relatives is not particularly high compared to genetic disorders in which a *single gene* determines whether someone develops the disease, such as cystic fibrosis or Huntington disease, where the increased risk to a first-degree relative is 1,000 to 10,000-fold higher than the risk of disease in the general population. In fact, the increased risk of TS for a close relative of a TS-affected individual is much more similar to the increased risk of heart disease or diabetes for a family member of a person with one of those conditions. This is because, although TS is highly genetic, it is probably not caused by a single gene, and therefore the chances are lower that any particular individual in a TS family will get the "right" combination of genes necessary to cause TS.

While most TS families only have a few family members with TS, a small number of families have been identified where TS is present in every generation and where many family members in each generation have TS or a related tic disorder. While these families are not typical or representative of the general TS population, their pattern of inheritance suggests that these families in particular may have a stronger genetic form of TS and thus may serve as guides in the search to identify underlying TS genes.

TS-RELATED CONDITIONS

Chronic Tics

Family studies indicate that chronic tic disorders (chronic motor tics only or chronic vocal tics only) occur more frequently in relatives of individuals with TS than in the general population. Specifically, approximately 10-20% of first-degree relatives of a person with TS will have chronic tics (CT) in addition to the 5-15% of first-degree relatives with TS[4]. Overall, these data suggest that the chance of a sibling or child of a TS-affected person having either TS or CT is about 15-30%, with the chance for boys being slightly higher than the chance for girls. As described in the section above, twin studies also support the idea that TS and CT are probably different manifestations of the same common underlying genetic factors.

Obsessive Compulsive Disorder (OCD)

OCD is in general a more commonly occurring disorder than TS, affecting approximately 2% of people worldwide. Current studies suggest that some forms of OCD may be genetically related to TS and CT, particularly when the three disorders run together in the same family. These studies are complicated by the fact that many people with TS will have OC-behaviors, which can sometimes be indistinguishable from complex motor tics. Nevertheless, in families with TS or CT, about 5-20% of first-degree relatives will have OC-behaviors or OCD in the absence of tics, with girls being more likely to have OC-behaviors and boys somewhat less likely[1,4]. At the same time, there are some families with OCD in which no family members have TS or other tic disorders. Currently, it is not known whether these families with OCD but no tics share overlapping genetic factors with TS and CT or whether their OCD has a different underlying set of genetic susceptibilities.

Attention Deficit Hyperactivity Disorder/Attention Deficit Disorder (ADHD/ADD)

ADHD (previously called ADD) is another fairly common disorder, occurring in about 6% of people in the US and worldwide. Like OCD, ADHD occurs more frequently than would be expected in people with TS based on the occurrence rates of ADHD in the general population. However, unlike OCD, where research strongly suggests that at least some forms of OCD and TS are genetically related, it is still not known whether ADHD and TS share common genetic factors. Current research shows that TS and ADHD often co-occur within the same individual in a family, but that ADHD is not necessarily more common among TS family members who do not have tics. The reasons for this unusual pattern of ADHD occurrence in TS families are still not clear, and the TS-ADHD relationship is an active area of scientific study.

An intriguing recent finding from a study of sibling pairs and parents with TS found that the combination of "TS plus ADHD and OCD" may represent a specific subtype of TS which in itself is "highly genetic"[5]. Future genetic research examining this combination of three conditions together may help to understand whether TS+OCD+ADHD is somehow different genetically from TS or CT alone or not.

TS INHERITANCE—THE BIG PICTURE

Early family studies of TS inheritance suggested that TS, CT and OCD might be transmitted from one family member to another by a single "TS gene". Under this assumption, an affected parent would pass on this gene to one or more of his/her children, and those children would then have an increased risk for developing TS. However, the studies above indicate that, for the vast majority of families, TS does not appear to be caused by problems in a single gene. Instead, researchers now believe that TS is much more complex, and may be caused by problems in a few genes or possibly tens to hundreds of genes working together within a family. If this is indeed the case, then, in order to find the relevant TS genes, TS genetics researchers will need to study very large numbers of individuals and families with TS to identify the many different "TS genes" and to understand how they combine to cause TS.

TS GENETIC STUDIES

While twin and family-based inheritance studies demonstrate that genetic factors are important in causing TS, these studies in themselves do not test for abnormalities in specific genes. Researchers have done many experiments searching for those specific genes using a variety of genetic approaches, though identifying any one gene as a "TS gene" with certainty has been challenging. So far, three genes have been identified that may explain the causes of TS in a small number of individual families[6-8]. These families have been studied either because there is a known genetic re-arrangement in a family member (known as a chromosomal translocation) or because an unusually large number of individuals in the family have TS. Two of these genes, *contactin associated protein-like 2* (CNTNAP2) and *SLIT and NTRK-like family, member 1* (SLITRK1), appear to be important in helping nerve cells form connections to other cells. The third gene, *histidine decarboxylase* (HDC), is a key enzyme in producing the transmitter histamine in the brain. Thus far, however, defects in two of these genes (CNTNAP2 and HDC) have been found only in one family each, and mutations in SLITTRK1 have been limited to fewer than 10 individuals with TS. Because these genes affect only a very few families, they are not currently useful for genetic testing to decide whether someone is at risk for TS, nor are they currently helpful in deciding how to treat TS. Nonetheless, these discoveries are still critically important, since they provide insight into what kinds of genes may be altered in TS, which could help to identify more TS genes and could open up new avenues of research into TS treatments. For example, if genetic researchers look at other genes that are known to interact biologically with these 3 genes, they may find differences in these interacting genes in other individuals with TS. If that turns out to be the case, scientists may be able to string together an underlying biological mechanism by which different genes work together to cause TS. This is one area of active current research.

In another approach, TS researchers have gathered together large families where TS or CT is present in many individuals throughout each family (ranging from 5 to 94 TS–or CT-affected individuals per family). They have studied these families with genetic markers spread throughout the human genome to look for specific genetic regions that are shared between relatives with TS or CT in each family. These efforts have identified a region on chromosome 2 that appears to harbor at least one TS gene, and two additional regions on chromosomes 6 and 17 that may also contain TS genes[9]. Efforts to study these families further, with finer scale genetic mapping as well as sequencing of these chromosomal regions, are underway and may provide additional TS genes in the near future.

Lastly, TS scientists have been looking at hundreds or thousands of individuals with TS, either alone or together with their parents, to try to identify TS genes. Some of these studies involve looking at over 500,000 single changes in DNA that are common in the general population to identify those changes that occur more often in people with TS than in people without TS (these studies are known as genome-wide association studies). Other studies search for stretches of DNA where there are too many or too few copies (that are either duplicated or deleted) in individuals with TS. These studies are known as copy number variant (CNV) studies, and have been successful in identifying genes for complex neuropsychiatric disorders like autism. Both of these types of studies have been undertaken recently in TS and results are expected to be reported in the near future.

NON-GENETIC CONTRIBUTIONS

Although genetic factors clearly contribute to the development of TS and other tic disorders, genes are not the entire story. As discussed previously, twin and family studies have suggested that additional, non-genetic factors are also important in the development of TS and other tic disorders. Such factors are also probably responsible for the wide range of symptoms seen between individuals, including when the symptoms start, the severity of the symptoms, and the development of co-occurring disorders such as OCD and ADHD. Studies of non-genetic factors (also called "environmental factors") in TS have primarily focused on stressful and other events during the pre-natal (prior to birth), perinatal (during birth), or early life periods, particularly those which could potentially cause damage to the developing brain. These studies have examined factors such as the mother's use of tobacco, alcohol, drugs, prescribed medication, or caffeine during her pregnancy or birth. Also, studies have looked at pregnancy complications such as low oxygen at birth, excessive vomiting during pregnancy, low birth weight, or the umbilical cord wrapped around the baby's neck at birth and the level of the mother's anxiety or stress during her pregnancy[10].

Environmental risk factors such as those listed above are thought to interact with TS genes by affecting how the genes are expressed, possibly by causing these genes to be turned on or off inappropriately, or by influencing the level of expression of the genes such that they are expressed at higher or lower rates than normal during pregnancy and childhood.

There are still only a few studies of the relationship between non-genetic/environmental factors and TS, and these studies are complicated by the fact that most of them use information collected from parents or medical records years after the child's birth. Partly for this reason, the results of the studies are not entirely consistent with each other. However, some patterns are beginning to emerge. Those non-genetic risk factors that have been the most studied are discussed below.

Birth Weight

Several studies have looked at the relationship between birth weight and TS, including twin studies, studies of individuals with TS compared to those without TS (such studies are called case-control studies), and studies looking at the relationship between birth weight and tic severity or the presence of OCD or ADHD. In the twin studies, which were relatively small due to the difficulty in finding twins with TS, the twin with TS or the twin with more severe symptoms had a lower birth weight than his/her unaffected or less severely affected co-twin[10]. However, in contrast to the findings in twins, a large study that looked at tic severity and the presence or absence of OCD and ADHD in unrelated individuals with TS found no relationship between tic severity and birth weight, but did find a relationship between lower birth weight and the presence of ADHD[11]. Another large study comparing children with "TS only" to children with TS plus ADHD also found lower birth weight in the children with TS and ADHD[12]. Additional studies though have not been able to find any relationship between lower birth weight and either the presence of TS, increased tic severity, or co-occurring OCD or ADHD.

Prenatal Maternal Smoking
Multiple studies have looked at the relationships between the mother's use of tobacco, alcohol, drugs, caffeine, or prescription medications with the development either of TS, tic severity, or of co-occurring OCD and ADHD. Use of caffeine and prescription medications have not consistently been shown to be associated with TS, tic severity, OCD or ADHD. Use of alcohol and/or drugs during pregnancy has been reported to be associated with increased risk of developing co-occurring OCD in one study, but other studies have not found this relationship. However, several studies have shown a relationship between mothers smoking during their pregnancies and either development of TS or increased tic severity in individuals with TS[10-11]. Similarly, several studies have shown an association between maternal smoking during pregnancy and co-occurring OCD or ADHD in children with TS[11-13]. While not all studies have been able to demonstrate these relationships, prenatal maternal smoking is now emerging as the most consistently identified environmental risk factor either for development of TS, or for increased severity of symptoms (including increased tic severity and increased risk of having co-occurring OCD and/or ADHD). Clearly, however, as most mothers do not smoke during their pregnancies, this is not the only environmental risk factor for TS; similarly, if smoking is a contributor to TS, it may only be a small piece of a much larger puzzle involving genes and other non-genetic factors.

Complications During Pregnancy/Delivery

Several studies have reported an association between complications during pregnancy and increased rates of TS or increased symptom severity in those with TS. Pregnancy complications include severe maternal nausea and vomiting during pregnancy (hyperemesis), severely high maternal blood pressure such that it threatens the fetus (pre-eclampsia), poor maternal health, advanced maternal age, gestational diabetes, and high risk of miscarriage, among other things. Delivery complications include traumatic or difficult delivery, use of forceps or vacuum suction to deliver the baby, emergent or urgent (unplanned) cesarean section, umbilical cord wrapped around the baby's neck, low oxygen (hypoxia) at birth, and similar complications. No pregnancy or delivery complication in particular has been consistently shown to be associated with an increased risk of TS or increased symptom severity. However, several studies have suggested that pregnancy and delivery complications when taken as a group may be associated with an increased risk of TS and an increased severity of TS symptoms, especially when more than one complication is present.

Psychological Stress

Psychological stress during pregnancy is difficult to study effectively, and, in particular, is difficult to accurately recall and quantify when asked about several years after the pregnancy. Therefore, most studies of environmental risk factors and TS have not examined the role of psychological stress. However, at least two studies have found an association between increased risk of TS, increased risk of TS plus ADHD, and/or increased severity of tic symptoms and severe psychological or emotional stress in the mother during her pregnancy[13]. More work needs to be done in this area, but the studies that have been done do suggest that psychosocial stress during pregnancy may be a contributing risk factor in TS.

CONCLUSION

Thirty years of research have now demonstrated convincingly that TS and CT have strong genetic influences, but it is also becoming clear that there is no single "TS gene", as previously thought. Instead, it appears that TS is inherited in a complex fashion, with many genes working together with other non-genetic factors to cause TS in each person. In addition, the specific "TS genes" are likely to be different in different individuals or families with TS. Similarly, possible environmental risk factors are now beginning to be identified; progress in this area will happen much more quickly once TS genes are found, and the role of specific environmental factors can be studied in people who carry TS risk genes and either do or do not develop TS. TS genetic researchers worldwide, using a variety of scientific approaches, are currently examining these questions with the goal of uncovering the underlying causes of TS in the relatively near future. Once a larger number of TS genes have been found, scientists can begin to study how these different genes interact with each other and with non-genetic risk factors to cause TS. Ultimately, this research should lead to a better understanding of the fundamental biological processes that cause TS and hopefully guide us towards new treatments aimed at lessening the symptoms of TS and related conditions.

References

1. O'Rourke, J.A., Scharf, J.M., Yu, D. & Pauls, D.L. (2009) The genetics of Tourette syndrome: a review. *J Psychosom Res* **67(6)**, 533-545.

2. Ooki, S., (2005) Genetic and environmental influences on stuttering and tics in Japanese twin children. *Twin Res Hum Genet* **8(1)**, 69-75.

3. Bolton, D., Rijsdijk, F., O'Connor, T.G., Perrin, S. & Eley, T.C. (2007) Obsessive-compulsive disorder, tics and anxiety in 6-year-old twins. *Psychol Med* **37(1)**, 39-48.

4. Scharf, J.M. & Pauls, D.L. (2007) Genetics of Tic Disorders. In: Rimoin DL, Connor JM, Pyeritz RE, Korf BR, eds. *Emery and Rimoin's Principles and Practices of Medical Genetics.* 5th ed. Churchill Livingstone/Elsevier, PA. pp. 2737-2754.

5. Grados, M.A. & Mathews, C,A. (2008) Latent class analysis of Gilles de la Tourette syndrome using comorbidities: clinical and genetic implications. *Biol Psychiatry* **64(3)**, 219-225.

6. Verkerk, A.J., Mathews, C.A., Joosse, M., Eussen, B.H., Heutink, P. & Oostra BA. (2003) CNTNAP2 is disrupted in a family with Gilles de la Tourette syndrome and obsessive compulsive disorder. *Genomics* **82(1)**, 1-9.

7. Abelson, J.F., Kwan, K.Y., O'Roak, B.J., Baek, D.Y., Stillman, A.A., Morgan, T.M., Mathews, C.A., Pauls, D.L., Rasin, M.R., Gunel, M., Davis, N.R., Ercan-Sencicek, A.G., Guez, D.H., Spertus, J.A., Leckman, J.F., Dure, L.S. 4th, Kurlan, R., Singer, H.S., Gilbert, D.L., Farhi, A., Louvi, A., Lifton, R.P., Sestan, N. & State, M.W. (2005) Sequence variants in SLITRK1 are associated with Tourette's syndrome. *Science* **310(5746)**, 317-320.

8. Ercan-Sencicek, A.G., Stillman, A.A., Ghosh, A.K., Bilguvar, K., O'Roak, B.J., Mason, C.E., Abbott, T., Gupta, A., King, R.A., Pauls, D.L., Tischfield, J.A., Heiman, G.A., Singer, H.S., Gilbert, D.L., Hoekstra, P.J., Morgan, T.M., Loring, E., Yasuno, K., Fernandez, T., Sanders, S., Louvi, A., Cho, J.H., Mane, S., Colangelo, C.M., Biederer, T., Lifton, R.P., Gunel, M. & State, M.W. (2010) L-histidine decarboxylase and Tourette's syndrome. *N Engl J Med* **362(20)**, 1901-1908.

9.   TSAICG. (2007) Genome scan for Tourette disorder in affected-sibling-pair and multigenerational families. *Am J Hum Genet* **80(2),** 265-272.

10. Walkup, J.T. (2001) Epigenetic and environmental risk factors in Tourette syndrome. *Adv Neurol* **85,** 273-279.

11. Mathews, C.A., Bimson, B., Lowe, T.L., Herrera, L.D., Budman, C.L., Erenberg, G., Naarden, A., Bruun, R.D., Freimer, N.B. & Reud, V.I. (2006) Association between maternal smoking and increased symptom severity in Tourette's syndrome. *Am J Psychiatry* **163(6),** 1066-1073.

12. Pringsheim, T., Sandor, P., Lang, A., Shah, P. & O'Connor, P. (2009) Prenatal and perinatal morbidity in children with Tourette syndrome and attention-deficit hyperactivity disorder. *J Dev Behav Pediatr* **30(2),** 115-121.

13. Motlagh, M.G., Katsovich, L., Thompson, N., Lin, H., Kim, Y.S., Scahill, L., Lombroso, P.J., King, R.A., Peterson, B.J. & Leckman, J.F. (2010) Severe psychosocial stress and heavy cigarette smoking during pregnancy: an examination of the pre- and perinatal risk factors associated with ADHD and Tourette syndrome. *Eur Child Adolesc Psychiatry* **19(10),** 755-764.

Glossary

Chromosome: A single, long molecule of DNA (ranging in size from 50-250 million bases of DNA) that is observable as a condensed strand when examined under a microscope. Each human cell typically has 46 chromosomes, 23 of which are inherited from a child's mother and 23 from his/her father.

DNA: Abbreviation for deoxyribonucleic acid, the chemical material inside cells that contains coded genetic information. DNA consists of four different "bases" (A, C, G, T) that are arranged in an ordered sequence which when read by cellular machinery provides the instructions that direct cell function.

Environmental Risk Factor: The general term for any contributor to disease risk that is "not genetic". It is important to note that not all environmental risk factors are truly "environmental", i.e. caused by exposures in the environment. For example, gender is commonly considered an "environmental" risk factor for many conditions.

Family study: A type of genetic study in which relatives of an individual with a genetic condition are examined to determine how often the condition occurs in family members as well as the specific pattern of recurrence throughout the family.

First-degree relative: A family member who shares 50% of their DNA with another family member. This includes parents, children and siblings.

Gene: A stretch of DNA sequence that forms a functional unit which influences a particular trait (like eye color or height) or a medical condition.

Genome: The complete set of genes in each cell of the body. The human genome is currently thought to contain 20,000-25,000 genes.

Inheritance: The pattern by which a condition is passed down through families. The degree to which a condition is genetic is also called its "heritability".

Mutation: An alteration in the underlying DNA sequence of a gene that changes the gene's normal function.

Twin study: A type of genetic study in which the presence of a specific condition is compared between identical and non-identical (fraternal) twins to estimate the degree to which the condition under study is due to genetic factors.

CHAPTER 8

PEDIATRIC AUTOIMMUNE NEUROPSYCHIATRIC DISORDERS ASSOCIATED WITH STREPTOCOCCAL INFECTION (PANDAS) AND TOURETTE SYNDROME

Tanya Murphy, M.D., M.S.

INTRODUCTION

Pediatric Autoimmune Neuropsychiatric Disorders Associated with Streptococcus (PANDAS) is a subtype of childhood onset Obsessive Compulsive Disorder (OCD) and tic disorders, first described over 10 years ago. The possibility that Group A Streptococcus (GAS) infections can play a role in triggering tics and OCD in some children has gained support but has not yet been proven. Linking the onset of neuropsychiatric symptoms to infection would certainly explain the dramatic changes that have been described in these previously healthy children. This chapter provides an overview of the current scientific and clinical impression of an area where unfortunately, too little is known and controversy is high about the existence, characteristics, diagnostic boundaries and treatment of PANDAS.

CHARACTERISTICS OF PANDAS

Typically, children will have a sudden, dramatic onset or worsening of tics, excessive worrying, obsessive and/or compulsive behaviors. Symptoms occur before puberty with an average onset age of less than 7 years. This dramatic change occurs in association with or following a 'strep throat' infection. Classically, high functioning and well-adjusted children will change before their parents' eyes in a matter of 24-72 hours with a range of psychiatric symptoms (e.g. increased irritability, frequent mood and personality changes, rage episodes, anxiety, hyperactivity, and oppositional behaviors). These behaviors often cause significant disruption of family, social, and school functioning.

Other associated symptoms reported by parents include a deterioration of handwriting skill (big, sloppier letters—see figures 1-4), poor academic performance (particularly math skills), a decrease in motor skills, as well as onset of inattentiveness, frequent urination, and nightmares. Academic decline and difficulty with attention and learning tasks are common and are usually seen in most PANDAS children, even those without an Attention Deficient Hyperactivity Disorder diagnosis. Comorbid conditions or symptoms describe any other disorders or symptoms that are present in addition to tics and OCD as part of the PANDAS diagnosis. ADHD, Oppositional Defiant Disorder, Major Depressive Disorder, separation anxiety, and learning disabilities are among the most common comorbid disorders in PANDAS children. These disorders are also very common in tics and OCD that present in the usual manner. However, with children that best fit a PANDAS presentation, the primary difference is that the symptoms of these disorders (mood disturbance, hyperactivity, oppositional behaviors, etc.) present at or near the time of the tic/OCD onset and it is not unusual for the child to have symptoms of all of these disorders develop at the same time.

PANDAS CRITERIA (National Institutes of Mental Health)

• The presence of OCD and/or tic disorder
• Pediatric onset of symptoms (ages 3 years to puberty)
• Episodic course of symptom severity
• A temporal association between symptom onset and infection

- Presence of mild neurological abnormalities (hyperactivity, choreiform movements, handwriting deterioration)
- *No evidence of chorea, rheumatic carditis or arthritis

*not a formal criterion but assumed

ASSOCIATED SYMPTOMS
- Frequent urination
- Frequent upper respiratory infections (cough, sinusitis, ear infections), strep throat, etc., prior to the age of 7
- History of behavioral improvement on antibiotics
- History of tonsillectomy/adenoidectomy
- High streptococcal titers
- Frequent but non-specific findings include: Family history of autoimmune disorder, separation anxiety, meltdowns, eating fears (choking or contaminated food), difficulty copying from the board, and a new onset of bedwetting

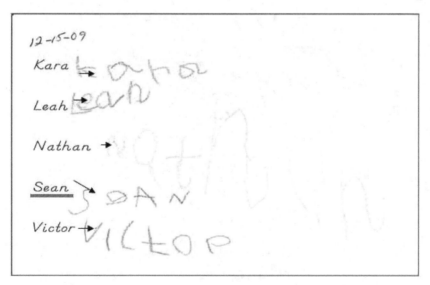

Figure 1. Five year old before the onset of OCD/tics.

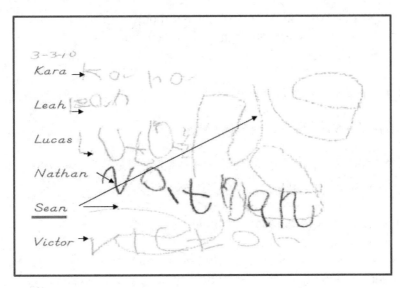

Figure 2. The same boy three months later.

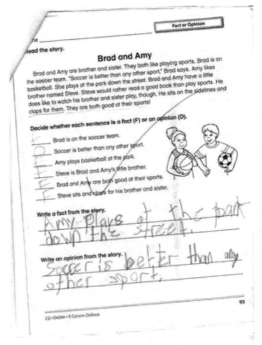

Figure 3. Nine year old boy with OCD and tics (PANDAS) Pre Treatment-assignment took nearly one hour with a struggle and tears.

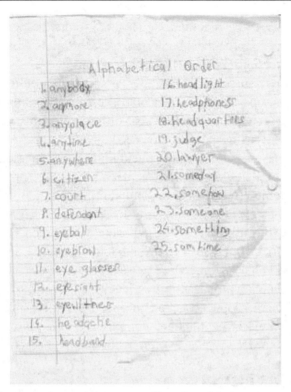

Figure 4. The same boy, after three weeks of antibiotic therapy, finished this assignment in a few minutes without difficulty.

TRIGGERS

While PANDAS is not a contagious disease, GAS is highly contagious through direct person-to-person contact. In PANDAS, these streptococcal infections are thought to create a cascade of immune and autoimmune events in children most susceptible: children ages 5-15 years old. GAS infections are responsible for a wide range of illnesses, from common mild sore throats and skin infections (impetigo) to rare serious diseases such as rheumatic fever (inflammation of the heart valves) and acute glomerulonephritis (a kidney condition). Typical symptoms in streptococcal pharyngitis include sore throat, fever, and swollen tonsils and lymph nodes. Younger children may experience abdominal pain, nausea, and vomiting or perineal/vaginal redness. Although these symptoms are uncomfortable and the illness is contagious, the primary reason for treating with antibiotics is to prevent illnesses like rheumatic fever that are due to an autoimmune reaction to the streptococcal bacteria.

Other infectious agents (mycoplasma, influenza, Lyme disease) have also been suspected to trigger a sudden onset of OCD, tics and other neuropsychiatric disorders. Typical symptoms of viral or bacterial infections that would present differently than strep throat are the presence of runny nose and/or a cough. A common presentation of a mycoplasma infection is pneumonia, often called "walking pneumonia" for its milder symptoms that rarely require hospitalization. School aged children often have minimal or no symptoms at all. When infections do occur, it is important to treat the infection promptly and completely with antibiotics. Close exposure to streptococcus via family members or friends may also contribute to the presence of tic flare ups or an unexpected lack of response to treatment. Symptom exacerbation commonly begins within one to two weeks following the infection or immune trigger. In some cases, parents seem to 'know' that their child is getting ill by observing the flare up in the child's tics, anxiety or OCD that occurs before the typical symptoms of an infection have begun.

IMMUNIZATIONS

Immunizations are an important factor in acquiring immunity to several infectious agents that are known to trigger PANDAS symptoms. Immunizations should ideally be given when a child is not ill. Some children do have exacerbations following vaccinations; however, by building immunity to common triggers, the longer-term outcome could be a reduction in symptom severity. Exacerbations following immunizations are generally shorter and less severe than those accompanied by the actual illnesses such as influenza A.

COURSE OF SYMPTOMS

Children with PANDAS have a sudden onset or worsening of their symptoms, often described as happening "overnight." This onset of symptoms may include motor and vocal tics, which are clearly different from that of a simple tic. Children in the PANDAS subgroup will experience a cluster of simultaneous motor and vocal tics with greater frequency and intensity than that of a typical tic onset. The onset of OCD symptoms in these children is also clearly distinguished from a non-PANDAS related onset; symptoms can be clinically impairing in

24-48 hours[3]. Parents will describe that their child completely 'changed' overnight in temperament and personality.

The precise factors associated with whether PANDAS remits or progresses to a more chronic illness like TS have not been established. The course of OCD and tic symptoms in PANDAS typically has a 'sawtooth' or remitting course with varying characteristics dependent on the child's gender, age, comorbidity, and illness duration[2]. These exacerbations often will diminish significantly over time or even resolve completely in six to eight weeks. Subsequent exacerbations may occur with increased severity and impairment and persist for several weeks[1]. For many others, symptoms may never reappear and will resemble the tic diagnosis of Transient Tic Disorder.

EVALUATION AND DIAGNOSIS

Clinical History Is Very Important

Although there is no "PANDAS test", the medical history of the child is very important. For example: Does the child have a history of frequent, repeated infections, scarlet fever (rash reaction that accompanies streptococcal infections), previous but brief episodes of tics, OCD, or compulsive urination? Was the onset of anxiety, OCD, and tics very dramatic and very severe within a time span of 1-2 days? Were there exposures to others that had been ill? These are questions that must be answered to make an accurate diagnosis of PANDAS.

Throat Cultures

For children with new onset symptoms, a throat culture will provide useful information; especially if it is positive (meaning a current infection was detected). Treatment of the throat infection may lead to tic or OCD improvement. Many clinics use "rapid strep tests" and when positive, this result is enough to confirm a streptococcal infection. If negative, it should ideally be followed with a 24-48 hour culture.

Streptococcal Antibody Tests

This type of testing requires a blood draw, which aims to detect antibodies (immune response) to previous streptococcal infections. The levels of these antibodies are sometimes called titers. Commonly used antibodies in commercial laboratories are anti-streptolysin O and anti-deoxyribonuclease B. The anti-streptolysin O is more specific to throat infections and the anti-DNase B shows a strong response to streptococcal skin infections (e.g. Impetigo). The presence of elevated streptococcal antibody titers can confirm the presence of an immune response to streptococcus at some time point but as a stand-alone test, it does not confirm a PANDAS diagnosis. While elevation in these antibodies are commonly found in children with PANDAS presentations, careful consideration of the clinical history and examination of the child is also required. In some cases, particularly for very young children, antibodies may not be elevated due to lack of enough prior exposures to meet laboratory thresholds especially if they are not age adjusted. Many factors may influence a single time point measure of streptococcal antibodies. The time from infection to the time the sample is drawn certainly has high variability in a clinical population and will affect values obtained. Other factors such as an individual's cholesterol level, treatment with antibiotics, and the individual's ability to mount a strong immune response are other potential reasons for variations in titer levels.

Normal Range of Streptococcal Titers		
	ASO Titer	**Anti-DNase B**
Adult	<160 Todd units/mL or <200 IU	<85 Todd units/mL
Child (5-12 years)	170-330 Todd units/mL	<170 Todd units/mL
Preschool-aged Child	100-160 Todd units/mL	<60 Todd units/mL

Ideally, whenever possible, obtaining streptococcal titers at symptom onset of <2 weeks duration and again 3-6 weeks later will provide strong support of a streptococcal trigger if a fourfold rise in titers is observed. In children with symptom onset exceeding four weeks before examination, streptococcal titers will add support but not provide proof that tic or OCD symptoms resulted from a streptococcal infection. Other clinical factors like the acute and severe onset of tics and OCD will need to be considered as well.

Also, it is important to point out that elevations of these antibodies do not mean that the child has a current/active streptococcal infection.

It may mean that the infection occurred at some time point weeks to months earlier. Elevated titers are also observed as a normal, healthy response to fighting off an infection. These antibodies can remain in the body after the infection is gone; but the amount of time these antibodies persist varies greatly between individuals. Many grade-school aged children can have chronically elevated titers (over months and years) without any medical consequences. Some children are also "strep carriers", whereas they have a positive culture without symptoms of infection. Children with mild immune deficiencies are at greater risk for recurrent infections including recurrent streptococcal infections leading to frequent observations of high titers.

Consultations

Depending on the presentation of the symptoms, various pediatric specialists may need to be involved, such as psychiatrists, neurologists, cardiologists, rheumatologists, infectious disease/immunologists, and psychologists. For example, a child with a very severe sudden onset of anxiety, tics, and coordination loss should be assessed by a pediatrician for consideration of the need to refer the child to a cardiologist to rule out carditis, or a neurologist to rule out other causes of loss of coordination.

TREATMENT

Standard Therapies

These children should continue to receive the standard care for patients with OCD and TS, including medications (e.g. guanfacine, aripiprazole, and fluoxetine in lower than typical starting doses) and therapies such as cognitive-behavioral therapy (CBT) and Habit Reversal Therapy. Until better guidelines are developed, children in the PANDAS subgroup should benefit from these evidence based treatments that may lessen the severity of a future flare up. OCD symptoms are best treated with CBT unless too severe to engage in therapy. CBT can help children remodel automatic responses to obsessions, teach skills that should prove helpful if symptoms do recur and also help families with behavioral strategies to lessen the risk of disrupted functioning and accommodation. Children often report feeling empowered from coping, relaxation, and resiliency skills learned in CBT. Antidepressants approved for OCD can also work well when started on a low dose (e.g., sertraline at 6.25 mg) that can be gradually increased as tolerated, but many of these children are sensitive to typical starting doses. Patients with tics respond well to a variety of evidence based pharmacologic agents and behavioral treatments if needed due to symptom severity and impairment.

Immune Based Treatments

Antimicrobial or immune based treatment of PANDAS should be based on each child's specific presentation. Children with symptoms of streptococcal infection should be tested and treated appropriately, typically with antibiotics, while being mindful that sometimes streptococcal infections can occur without complaint of a sore throat. Some strains of GAS are resistant to a certain class of antibiotics, the macrolides, and another type of antibiotic may be necessary in areas known to have resistant GAS. Anecdotally and supported in case studies, some children have dramatic improvements in tic/OCD symptoms and/ or behavior following standard antibiotic therapy. If a child continues to have frequent, recurrent infections and neuropsychiatric symptoms that coincide with the infections, family members should be tested using throat cultures to see if they are carriers and treated if shown to be positive. The optimal duration and dose of antibiotics needs to be formally studied. Prophylactic antibodies should only be considered if the history presents a strong association between repeated streptococcal infections and relapses. Clinical trials are currently underway to examine the effects of antibodies in these children.

Other treatments for PANDAS, such as plasmapheresis and intravenous immunoglobulin (IVIG) therapy, have been examined in research studies. The goal of plasmapheresis is to remove autoantibodies, that is, antibodies that are produced against the body's own tissues. This procedure involves removing the plasma, the fluid part of the blood, which contains these antibodies and replacing it with other fluids. Treatment takes several hours and can be done on an outpatient basis. An anticoagulant, medication to prevent blood clotting, is administered through the vein throughout this procedure. Common risks include a drop in blood pressure, experienced as dizziness, blurred vision, coldness, sweating or abdominal cramps. Other adverse effects include bleeding or allergic reactions.

IVIG is the infusion of immunoglobulins (antibodies) into the vein. This solution is composed of antibodies normally found in adult human blood that provide immunity against disease. IVIG products are derived from the plasma of a large number of individuals who have formed antibodies to a wide variety of bacteria, viruses, and other proteins. Plasma of all donors goes through several extensive screenings and testing for safety. The most common side effects include chills, low-grade fever, and headache. Rare serious side effects such as difficulty breathing, chest pain, seizures and severe anaphylactic reactions have been reported. Plasmapheresis and IVIG therapy are sometimes helpful for many immunological disorders, yet have not been proven safe and effective in PANDAS and are not recommended outside of research settings (check for current studies at National Institute of Mental Health (NIMH)). Immune therapies should be considered only if severely impaired and if conventional treatments or other less invasive treatments (e.g. trial of antibiotics) fail.

General Health
In some children, fine motor skills and less often, gross motor skills decline during the onset or marked flare ups of tics, anxiety or OCD. These losses are often temporary but some children will need evaluation by a neurologist to rule out other neurological problems and to be evaluated and treated by occupational or physical therapists to regain their baseline level of functioning.

Good health practices that decrease the potential of a pro-inflammatory state such as exercise, monitoring stress, and a healthy diet (e.g. a diet low in refined sugars, omega 6 and 9 fatty acids) may improve general health and improve resilience.

SCHOOL ACCOMMODATIONS
An individualized approach would best benefit the child. Many children benefit from an Individualized Education Program (IEP), with the child's academic needs as the focus that can also be modified as often as needed. Symptoms that are part of a PANDAS presentation, such as tics, anxiety, fine motor skill difficulty, and OCD may substantially reduce a child's ability to learn in the classroom. Proper documentation of difficulties relating to these symptoms and the child's ability to meet academic goals will be required to be eligible for a 504 plan.

The educational link found at www.tsa-usa.org is an excellent resource for clinicians, parents and educators. A range of necessary documents varies from school districts and schools may even require testing of their own. Accommodations may be used, but are not limited to include: untimed or extended time on tests or assignments, preferential seating to decrease embarrassment of tics, frequent breaks, and behavior intervention plans. As children with PANDAS often fluctuate in ability to focus, fine motor skills, and tolerance to sensory stimulation, the need for a certain level of accommodation may need more frequent adjustments than a child with typical ADHD or dyslexia. Children can greatly benefit from individualized accommodations, working towards their overall academic goals. Overall, a supportive school environment may alleviate possible triggers of exacerbation.

CONCLUSION

Although PANDAS is not currently listed as an official diagnosis in the Diagnostic and Statistical Manual of Mental Disorders, Fourth Edition or the International Classification of Diseases, Tenth Edition, the topic is a rapid-moving area of research in the medical field. Emerging evidence on PANDAS symptoms, course, and treatment should provide physicians, researchers, and parents a better understanding of what this clinical presentation involves. The phenomenon of PANDAS has continued to be met with interest and controversy concerning the association of infections with the dramatic onset of pediatric neuropsychiatric symptoms in a subgroup of children. The role of these infections has not been clearly defined; and additional research is required to determine the infectious association and treatment effectiveness for this group of children.

Acknowledgement: Leah Jung for her assistance.

References

1. Murphy, T., Kurlan, R. & Leckman, J. (2010). The Immunobiology of Tourette's Disorder, Pediatric Autoimmune Neuropsychiatric Disorders Associated with Streptococcus, and Related Disorders: A Way Forward. *J Child Adolesc Psychopharmacol* **20(4)**, 317-331.
2. Murphy, T., Sajid, M., Soto, O., Shapira, N., Edge, P., Yang, M., Lewis, M.H. & Goodman, W.K. (2004) Detecting pediatric autoimmune neuropsychiatric disorders associated with streptococcus in children with obsessive-compulsive disorder and tics. *Biol Psychiatry* **55(1)**, 61-68.
3. Swedo, S.E., Leonard, H.L. & Rapoport, J.L. (2004) The pediatric autoimmune neuropsychiatric disorders associated with streptococcal infection (PANDAS) subgroup: separating fact from fiction. *Pediatrics* **113(4)**, 907-911.
4. **http://www.nimh.nih.gov/about/director/index-ocd.shtml**

Glossary

Immunoglobulins: antibodies, proteins that are part of the immune response, increase to provide immunity to infections and sometimes are produced against the individuals tissues such as in autoimmune disorders (when antibodies are produced that do both, this can lead to an autoimmune response called molecular mimicry).

Strep throat, streptococcal tonsillitis, streptococcal pharyngitis: throat infections caused by Group A streptococcus

Titers: Antibody levels

CHAPTER 9

DRUG TREATMENTS FOR TOURETTE SYNDROME AND CO-MORBID DISORDERS

Donald L. Gilbert, M.D., M.S.

INTRODUCTION

There are three main objectives of this chapter: First, to provide a framework for thinking about when treatment with medications is a reasonable choice for managing TS associated symptoms, primarily tics, ADHD (Attention Deficit Hyperactivity Disorder), and OCD (Obsessive Compulsive Disorder) symptoms. Second, to provide a framework for evaluating claims in medical literature and the internet, that a particular medication or other intervention is useful for treating TS. Finally, to provide a brief account of medical treatments currently used for tics, as well as ADHD and OCD for persons with TS.

WHEN TO TREAT TS SYMPTOMS WITH BRAIN MEDICATION

The decision to start a medical treatment for yourself, your child, or other family member is not to be taken lightly. As doctors who treat hundreds and hundreds of children and adults with TS, we would like to provide some general background, based on observations we have made in TS clinics.

1. Some patients go to see TS specialists while taking high doses of medication despite having relatively minor tics like head shaking. Sometimes children as young as 3 or 4 years old are taking medications because the parents are upset by symptoms, despite the fact that their symptoms are not interfering with the child's life. Other patients with much more obvious or frequent tics do not want medication. Thus, the tic-related impairment and decisions about medication often do not seem to correlate well with the actual need for therapy.

2. For many patients, the symptoms necessary to make the diagnosis of TS, the tics, are the mildest problem. ADHD, OCD, problems with social skills, or anger can cause much more distress.

3. Some persons with TS think of it as a disease for which a cure is needed. At the present time, there is no cure for TS. Perhaps one day, if the cause or causes of TS become known, a cure may be possible.

4. Some individuals seem to consider TS as a part of them, that may flare up, but that does not need treatment most of the time. These persons seem a bit more at peace with the diagnosis, and do not want to take any medicine that would change their personality or risk any harm. Although the definitions of Disease and Disorder are a little imprecise, and experts may use these terms interchangeably, disorders, conditions like ADHD, depression, migraines, many forms of epilepsy, and TS, do not involve death of brain cells. Rather, these conditions involve changes in the way brain cells communicate with one another. They may or may not cause life interference, but fundamentally they can't be fully "fixed".

The approach doctors take when making decisions about treating tics, ADHD, OCD, etc., are very similar to decisions about treating other conditions of the brain, like tremor, as well as symptoms outside the brain, like runny noses and itchy eyes from allergies. To summarize:

The emphasis should be on whether symptoms interfere with the quality of life. For tics, problems can include pain, functional interference, social embarrassment, and classroom or work disruption. If the symptoms are not disruptive in any way, they do not need to be treated. In such cases, treatment risks likely outweigh potential benefits. The focus of medical treatment should be on the person taking the medication. The fact that a person's tics upset a parent, a spouse, or another person is not a reason to treat. The association of tics with ADHD, OCD, or other cognitive or emotional problems is very common. It is important to rank symptoms in terms of severity and impairment before deciding which to treat. If treating medically, the goal is the safest treatment that improves symptoms without causing bothersome side effects. Success may be defined as reducing symptoms to a tolerable, manageable level.

MEDICATIONS: HOW DO WE KNOW SOMETHING WILL WORK? THE SCIENCE BEHIND HELPING PATIENTS

Medications can eradicate some conditions, like infections, and these results can be accurately measured. For example, if a patient has "strep throat," the doctor can reliably identify that the bacteria is present and, after antibiotic treatment, can reliably identify that it is gone. In treating a disease that is fatal, medications that reduce the death rate or prolong the average life span can usually be reliably identified. Medications can temporarily eliminate some brain disturbances. For example, some individuals with milder forms of epilepsy can be completely seizure free after taking the right anti-seizure medication (although if they stop the medicine, the seizures may return). However, behaviors and thoughts such as tics, obsessions, impulsive tendencies, are much harder to objectively measure and eliminate. As a rule, medications cannot eliminate relatively normal behaviors that are simply performed excessively. For example:

- **Blinking tics**: Everyone blinks. Medications are not going to eliminate blinking tics unless you completely paralyze the blinking apparatus. But that's no good-blinking serves a useful purpose!
- **Obsessions**: Everyone worries—and worrying can be a good thing. You cannot completely eliminate obsessions and worries, unless you completely inhibit worrying. Then you have someone who is apathetic and doesn't care about anything—and that's not good either!

- **Impulsivity**: Everyone acts impulsively from time to time. You cannot completely eliminate impulsivity unless you completely block motivation. Then you have someone who is a passive zombie—and that's not what you want either!

So if you can't cure it, and results are hard to measure, how do you know if a medication really works? This is a complex question that requires really going into depth on levels of scientific evidence. A few general guideposts for understanding what studies mean are described below in Table 1. Scientific studies lead to higher or lower degrees of confidence, but not absolute truths or certainty. As shown in figure 1, it is important to think about the type and quality of research and where the results put us on a spectrum between Definitely True and Definitely False.

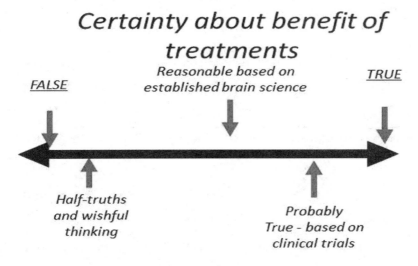

Figure 1. Schematic of Certainty

Table 1: General Guideposts for Understanding What Studies Mean

Important Features of Studies	Example
Studies reporting benefit in a small number of patients	Surgery for tics or OCD may look dramatically successful on TV, but if only a handful of patients have had a procedure, would you want to be the next person? If you are desperate enough to try a dramatic intervention that has only been tried in a few people, make sure you get several expert opinions and that you do it with an experienced, responsible group of physicians or as part of a careful research protocol. Small studies may not give accurate information about rare but important or life threatening side effects.
Open label studies	"Open label" studies are the classic example. In this type of study, everyone gets the medicine, and the doctors and the patients all know this. In this kind of study, a whole variety of explanations, including "the placebo effect," may be responsible for the apparent improvement. Careful studies done later often show the medicine does not work at all, or only has small benefits.
Randomized controlled trials comparing medicine to placebo	These are the most scientifically careful—and the least likely to be incorrect about benefit. A good sized study of 100 or more patients, where half the patients receive the medication and half receive placebo, and no one knows until the end who received which, is the most careful study design. If a medicine appears to work in this kind of study, most likely it really does work. Unfortunately, such studies are rarely done in TS, and often they involve groups of patients with tics but no other problems like OCD or ADHD.

Table 1: General Guideposts for Understanding What Studies Mean continued

"Statistically Significant" study results	You need to look at what the outcome was, how it was rated or measured, for how long, and was the effect important. For example, if a medication reduces symptoms by 25%, and a placebo pill "reduces" symptoms by 10%, is this difference enough to make the medication worth bothering with?
Studies in low profile journals your doctor has never heard of	Examples of high profile medical journals in the United States include JAMA and the New England Journal of Medicine. Most medical specialties, like neurology or psychiatry, have a few high impact journals as well. These journals review very carefully and reject most articles that are submitted to them for publication. You can usually trust results in these journals.
Studies showing remarkable benefit that are unpublished, only on the internet, or are found in journals you have never heard of are most likely not trustworthy	There is really no reason not to publish a good result unless you don't want careful scrutiny. There is no conspiracy to keep good treatments off the market. If something sounds too good to be true, at the time of this writing, it probably is.
Testimonials	Testimonials are a lot more persuasive to many people than statistics and science. If treatment comes with lots of testimonies, beware, because this weak form of evidence is a favorite technique of scam artists.
Biological plausibility	A favorite trick of purveyors of false treatments is to have a big section on their webpages about brain science. This makes them look smart and inspires some trust in readers. However, closer scrutiny usually reveals the fallacies in their reasoning. That said, it is important to point out that doctors will make decisions based on scientific knowledge about treatment in areas where direct evidence is still limited. Doctors spend years studying and gaining direct experience with the human body and diseases in order to acquire this knowledge. This is not the same as learning by surfing the internet.

MEDICATIONS: WHAT WORKS, HOW DOES IT WORK, AND HOW GOOD IS THE EVIDENCE?

In general, medicines act on systems within the brain that are used for communication between nerve cells (neurons). Some medicines act directly on the surface of brain cells, blocking or enhancing nerve firing. More commonly for TS, medicines act on chemicals that neurons release, called neurotransmitters. Medicines may increase, decrease, or stabilize the release of neurotransmitters. Alternatively, medicines may act in a way that mimics the brain's neurotransmitters and binds to their target's receptors. Binding to receptors can enhance, slow, or block signaling between brain cells.

Tics

Common medications used for treating tics are listed in Table 2. First line treatments for many physicians are clonidine and guanfacine, the alpha-2-adrenergic agonists. These are chosen first primarily because of safety. Second line treatments may be a group of medicines which sometimes work but have not been well studied, or the dopamine receptor blockers, also known as either neuroleptics or antipsychotics. These powerful medicines may suppress tics the best, but the risk of side effects is higher and closer monitoring is needed.

Table 2: Summary of Information on Medications Used for TS

TICS

Generics	Brands	Type	How They Work	FDA Approved for Tics	Studied Scienti- fically	In More Than 100 Patients	Main Side Effects	Other Comments
aripiprazole	Abilify	Dopamine receptor blocking agent which also may stabilize dopamine system and partly activate it	Blocking dopamine tends to reduce unwanted movements or thoughts	No	In progress	No	Weight gain, restlessness	
baclofen	Lioresal	GABA-B agonist	Acts on receptors that calm muscle spasm	No	Yes	No	Sedation	Used for spasticity
botulinum toxin injections into muscle	BOTOX	Blocks signaling from nerve to muscle	Slight weakening of the nerve motor connection or reducing the muscle strength seems to diminish the severity of a tic and reduce the urge to tic	No	No	No	Should be administered by experienced physician	Expensive; may not be covered by insurance
clonazepam	Klonopin	GABA-A agonist	Inhibits or slows brain activity in many areas	No	No	No	Too relaxing, sedating, has some addictive properties	Used for anxiety in adults
clonidine	Catapres oral but also patch	Alpha-2- adrenergic agonists	They bind to nerves that release norepinephrine, the "fight or flight" brain chemical and reduce its release, thereby probably allowing persons to remain calmer, more focused	No	Yes	Yes	Sleepiness, light headedness	First line for many years

Table 2: Summary of Information on Medications Used for TS
continued

Generics	Brands	Type	How They Work	FDA Approved for Tics	Studied Scientifically	In More Than 100 Patients	Main Side Effects	Other Comments
fluphenazine	Prolixin	Dopamine receptor blocking agent	Blocking dopamine tends to reduce unwanted movements or thoughts	No	No	No	Same as haloperidol	
guanfacine	Tenex, Intuniv	Alpha-2-adrenergic agonists	They bind to nerves that release norepinephrine, the "fight or flight" brain chemical and reduce its release, thereby probably allowing persons to remain calmer, more focused	No	Yes	No	Light headedness	Similar to clonidine but less sedating
haloperidol	Haldol	Dopamine receptor blocking agent	Blocking dopamine tends to reduce unwanted movements or thoughts	No	Yes	Yes	Unwanted weight gain, tremor, other neurologic side effects in short or long term, personality change, anxiety or school avoidance	First line for many years
pimozide	Orap	Dopamine receptor blocking agent	Blocking dopamine tends to reduce unwanted movements or thoughts	Yes	Yes	Yes	Same as haloperidol	Changes in heart rhythm
risperidone	Risperdal	Dopamine receptor blocking agent which also acts at serotonin receptors	Blocking dopamine tends to reduce unwanted movements or thoughts	No	Yes	Yes	Same as haloperidol, possibly more weight gain,	Although considered "atypical" it can still produce a lot of side effects similar to haloperidol

Table 2: Summary of Information on Medications Used for TS continued

Generics	Brands	Type	How They Work	FDA Approved for Tics	Studied Scienti- fically	In More Than 100 Patients	Main Side Effects	Other Comments
ropinirole	Requip	Dopamine agonist	Activates dopamine system but may also stabilize it	No	No	No	Sedation, nausea	Used for Restless Leg Syndrome, Parkinson's
tetrabenazine	Xenia	Dopamine receptor blocking agent which also acts "upstream" to reduce dopamine release	Blocking dopamine tends to reduce unwanted movements or thoughts	No	No	No	Lower risk of Tardive Dyskinesia	Recently FDA approved for Hunting- ton's disease, but not TS
topiramate	Topamax	Multi- mechanism anti-seizure medication	Complex effects on glutamate, pH of brain	No	Yes	No	Sedation, tingling, appetite suppression	Also used for migraine prevention

ADHD

A few commonly used medications used for treating ADHD are listed in Table 3. Stimulants are the most commonly used medications for treating ADHD symptoms. There are now a very large number of preparations in short and long acting forms. Most persons with TS plus ADHD can be treated as if they did not have tics. That is, the physician and patient/family can work toward optimizing ADHD treatments without worrying about making the tics worse in any meaningful way. Some persons with TS, particularly those with anxiety or who also have some autistic symptoms, are more likely to experience increased tics when taking prescribed stimulants. Non-stimulant options may also be used, and some of these are listed in the table as well. In TS, stimulants are often prescribed in conjunction with medications for tics and OCD. While most combinations have not been rigorously tested, they are in wide clinical use and can be beneficial. However, even if medications improve ADHD symptoms in childhood, there can still be major problems with academic underachievement and poor social outcomes in adolescence and adulthood.

Table 3: Summary of Information on Medications Used for ADD/ADHD

ADD/ADHD

Generics	Brands	Type	How They Work	FDA Approved for ADHD	Studied Scientifically	In More Than 100 Patients	Main Side Effects	Other Comments
amphetamine dextroamphetamine	Adderall, Dexedrine	Psycho-stimulants	Overall increase in release of dopamine and norepinephrine into front areas of brain needed for complex planning, attention, impulse regulation	No	Yes	Yes	Weight loss, appetite suppression, decreased vertical growth, insomnia, tics, tremor, personality change	A controlled substance with abuse potential. Usually first line treatment and well tolerated by children with tics
clonidine	Catapres oral but also skin patch	Alpha-2-adrenergic agonists	They bind to nerves that release norepinephrine, the "fight or flight" brain chemical and reduce its release, thereby probably allowing persons to remain calmer, more focused	No	Yes	Yes	Sleepiness, light headedness	Has been tested with methylphenidate
methylphenidate dexmethylphenidate	Ritalin, Concerta, Focalin, Methylin	Psycho-stimulants, oral but also patch	Overall increase in release of dopamine and norepinephrine into front areas of brain needed for complex planning, attention, impulse regulation	Yes	Yes	Yes	Weight loss, appetite suppression, decreased vertical growth, insomnia, tics, tremor, personality change	A controlled substance with abuse potential. Usually first line treatment and well tolerated by children with tics, has been tested with clonidine

Table 3: Summary of Information on Medications Used for ADD/ADHD continued

Generics	Brands	Type	How They Work	FDA Approved for ADHD	Studied Scientifically	In More Than 100 Patients	Main Side Effects	Other Comments
atomoxetine	Strattera	Norepine-phrine reuptake inhibitor	They bind to nerves that release norepinephrine and to a lesser extent dopamine, allowing these to act longer, thereby probably allowing persons to remain calmer, more focused	Yes	Yes	Yes	Appetite suppression, irritability, stomach upset	Has been tested in children with Tourette syndrome
guanfacine	Tenex, Intuniv	Alpha 2 adrenergic agonists	They bind to nerves that release norepinephrine, the "fight or flight" brain chemical and reduce its release, thereby probably allowing persons to remain calmer, more focused	No	Yes	Yes	Light headedness	Similar to clonidine but less sedating

OCD

Common medications used for treating OCD are listed in Table 4. Selective serotonin reuptake inhibitors are the most commonly used medication for treating OCD. Most testing of Selective Serotonin Reuptake Inhibitors for anxiety, OCD, or depression has been in adults. In adolescents, there has been recent concern that these medicines might induce suicidal thoughts. This discussion lies outside the scope of this chapter. However, it is well known that antidepressants can increase a person's energy level sooner than they improve negative thoughts. Thus, some individuals, shortly after starting anti-depressants, are at risk of acting on negative or aggressive thoughts that they are having toward themselves or others.

CONCLUSION

Treating TS is complicated and requires careful consideration of the variety of possible symptoms as well as impairment that these symptoms may cause for the person with the disorder. The scientific evidence for the benefit of medical treatments for TS symptoms is complex and needs to be interpreted cautiously by persons familiar with the research and principles of scientific study design. However, there are a number of medications available which, if prescribed carefully by experienced physicians, can reduce the burden of Tourette syndrome symptoms for many persons.

Table 4: Summary of Information on Medications Used for OCD

OCD

Generics	Brands	Type	How They Work	FDA Approved for OCD	Studied Scientifically	In More Than 100 Patients	Main Side Effects	Other Comments
citalopram	Celexa	Selective Serotonin Reuptake Inhibitor	By decreasing the reabsorption of serotonin by the nerve cells that release it, serotonin can act longer	No	Yes	Yes	Irritability, mania, apathy, sleep difficulties, tremor, nausea, withdrawal effects, suicidal ideation	
clomipramine	Anafranil	Tricyclic which is more selective for Serotonin Reuptake Inhibitor	By decreasing the reabsorption of serotonin by the nerve cells that release it, serotonin can act longer	No	Yes	Yes	Same as citalopram	More "anticholinergic" side effects
escitalopram	Lexapro	Selective Serotonin Reuptake Inhibitor	By decreasing the reabsorption of serotonin by the nerve cells that release it, serotonin can act longer	No	Yes	Yes	Same as citalopram	
fluoxetine	Prozac	Selective Serotonin Reuptake Inhibitor	By decreasing the reabsorption of serotonin by the nerve cells that release it, serotonin can act longer	No	Yes	Yes	Same as citalopram	
fluvoxamine	Luvox	Selective Serotonin Reuptake Inhibitor	By decreasing the reabsorption of serotonin by the nerve cells that release it, serotonin can act longer	No	Yes	Yes	Same as citalopram	

Table 4: Summary of Information on Medications Used for OCD continued

Generics	Brands	Type	How They Work	FDA Approved for OCD	Studied Scientifically	In More Than 100 Patients	Main Side Effects	Other Comments
paroxetine	Paxil	Selective Serotonin Reuptake Inhibitor	By decreasing the reabsorption of serotonin by the nerve cells that release it, serotonin can act longer	No	Yes	Yes	Same as citalopram	Has been tested in Tourette patients for rage
sertraline	Zoloft	Selective Serotonin Reuptake Inhibitor	By decreasing the reabsorption of serotonin by the nerve cells that release it, serotonin can act longer	No	Yes	Yes	Same as citalopram	Has been compared carefully to behavioral treatments and in combination with behavioral treatments for OCD

CHAPTER 10

TOURETTE SYNDROME, PREGNANCY AND BREASTFEEDING

Emilie R. Muelly, Ph.D. and Cheston M. Berlin Jr., M.D.

INTRODUCTION

The presence of a tic disorder, including TS, should not affect the course of a pregnancy. There is always concern about the effect on the fetus when there is maternal drug exposure. The literature concerning the possible effects of the medications used for TS and associated conditions is sparse and usually refers to the use of antidepressants and antipsychotics. There are very few drugs used during breast feeding that have an observable adverse effect on the infant; long term studies are needed for those medications affecting brain function.

PREGNANCY

Some women with TS may experience changes in their symptoms with pregnancy. However, experiences vary widely and our current knowledge does not allow us to predict the effects pregnancy will have on an individual woman's symptoms. In one survey with 63 female TS patient respondents, 9 of the 10 women who had been pregnant in the past did not report a change in tic frequency during or just following pregnancy[1]. In another study of eleven cases of pregnancy among eight female patients with TS, improvement in symptoms occurred in five of the pregnancies, worsening in three, and no effect in three[2]. Two of the mothers completed the pregnancies while taking haloperidol and fluoxetine. These infants were healthy. Of the three mothers that had two pregnancies evaluated for the study, the effects were the same for both pregnancies for a given mother.

LABOR & DELIVERY

It is unlikely that tics will create a problem in labor and delivery. In one case of a patient with severe tics, general anesthesia rather than regional anesthesia was used during a cesarean section to avoid the possibility of tics interfering with the procedure[3].

MEDICATIONS DURING PREGNANCY

Parents and medical professionals are concerned about the possible effects of exposure to drugs, alcohol, tobacco, and environmental chemicals during pregnancy. Although there are well known and publicized birth defects in infants whose mothers were exposed during pregnancy to drugs such as thalidomide and isotretenoin (Accutane®), the number of drugs that can cause obvious birth defects is fortunately quite small. Teratogen is the term given to any agent that produces a birth defect in a child if the exposure occurs during pregnancy. It is important to realize that a birth defect may be subtle and not immediately obvious in either the newborn period or during early infancy.

The best advice to expectant mothers is that they should avoid all medications when pregnant. The obstetrician may need to prescribe drugs for the well-being of the mother and infant, and she should follow this advice. Pregnant mothers should not use dietary supplements or herbal products because of difficulty in guaranteeing purity and safety for these compounds. Pregnant mothers should not smoke nor drink alcohol.

Many women with TS and other tic disorders can experience a lessening of tics during pregnancy. This may not occur for everyone, and tics are not the only symptom of a tic disorder for which medication is needed. The decision as to which medication and when to take it during a pregnancy is one which must be made by the patient and her physician. The purpose of this section is to provide information which may be helpful when such difficult decisions need to be made. If a decision is made to continue drug therapy, the dose should be as low as possible and treatment during the first trimester should be avoided.

TERATOGENS

Teratogens are agents which may produce birth defects in unborn children. A teratogen may be a drug, an environmental chemical, tobacco, alcohol, or radiation. Controversy exists over the role of other agents, examples of which are electromagnetic waves, certain foods and increased body temperature. A teratogen is most likely to have an effect on the human embryo during the first trimester (first 12 weeks) of a pregnancy. This is the time when the embryo is making many of the different body parts. During this period of time, some women may not realize that they are pregnant and may continue to be exposed to substances that may cause birth defects. Thus, it is important to address these concerns in advance if you are planning to become pregnant. If an unplanned pregnancy occurs, the mother should immediately seek the advice of her physician. Fetal ultrasound examinations and amniocentesis are tools available to assess the health of a fetus. The estimated baseline risk of fetal abnormality for all pregnancies is about 1 in 40 deliveries regardless of any exposures during pregnancy. Only a small fraction of these birth defects are attributed to a known exposure and many of these defects are minor.

A teratogen may also cause a defect that is not an obvious body defect, but may show itself as a problem in neurodevelopment as years pass by. In addition to these changes in body structure, there is the possibility of "behavioral teratogenesis". Exposure to these "behavioral teratogens" during pregnancy affects the developing brain, the effects from which may not be apparent until later in the child's life. This effect of pregnancy exposure may be in behavior and/or academic performance, especially in school. These neurological changes from "normal" may be subtle and difficult to detect. As variability in behavior or academic performance can have many causes, it is difficult to attribute any such change to exposure to any agent.

MEDICATIONS

Chapter 9 contains a thorough discussion of medications used in TS. This section contains a list of medications used in TS with some discussion as to their use during pregnancy. The following list is not meant to be comprehensive, but a list of the most commonly used drugs for the treatment of tics and other symptoms of TS. The chemical (generic) name is given first, followed by the trade name.

Antipsychotics are a common medication class used for tic suppression and include drugs such as haloperidol and risperidone. Generally they are not noted as significant agents for causing structural birth defects, particularly at doses prescribed for TS. However, if you are planning to become pregnant or have become pregnant, you should discuss with your physician whether or not adjustments should be made. Women taking any antipsychotic medication should receive 4 mg per day of folic acid because of the potential higher risk of neural tube defects[4].

Aripiprazole (Abilify®): There are only three case reports of this antipsychotic drug used during pregnancy[5-7]. Both were of women receiving higher doses for psychiatric diagnoses. One woman received the drug in the first 8 weeks, and again during week 20 only; another began the drug only in the 8th week of pregnancy, and a third during the last trimester. All three infants were normal.

Atomoxetine (Strattera®): This drug is a norepinepherine reuptake inhibitor used to treat Attention Deficit Hyperactivity Disorder (ADHD). There have not been many reports on the use of this drug during pregnancy. Three cases have been reported, two of which resulted in healthy newborns and one of which was lost to follow-up[8].

Clonazepam (Klonopin®): This tranquilizer is used for the treatment of anxiety and may be helpful for tic suppression. It is also used at higher doses as an anti-seizure medication. There are fewer than 100 case reports of use during pregnancy without concurrent use of other known teratogens, and few birth defects reported[9-11]. If taken throughout pregnancy, transient effect on neonatal behavior may be observed.

Clonidine (Catapres®; Kapvay®) and **Guanfacine** (Tenex®; Intuniv®): These two drugs are closely related and are alpha adrenergic agonists (act on the alpha receptors in the brain) and are used in some patients for symptoms of ADHD. There are no reports of fetal abnormalities after exposure to these drugs, despite their common use during pregnancy. Since these drugs were originally developed for the treatment of high blood pressure in adults, it would be prudent to monitor the newborn for changes in blood pressure.

Dextroamphetamine (Dexedrine®; Adderall®): These medications are used in treatment of ADHD. Abuse of amphetamines during pregnancy has been shown to increase risk of low birth weight, prematurity, and other complications. In a prospective study including 237 patients prescribed dextroamphetamine for weight control, continuation of the drug after 28 weeks of pregnancy in high weight females was associated with lower birth weight[12]. However, the decrease in birth weight was small and its clinical significance is not certain. In this and a similar study that included over 1500 patients taking dextroamphetamine clinically, no other complications and no malformations were reported to be in higher incidence than the control groups.

Fluphenazine (Prolixin®): There is no definite connection with exposure to this antipsychotic during pregnancy and birth defects. Rare single case reports described fetal abnormalities in women receiving this medication combined with other psychotropic drugs. Some cases have reported transit changes in behavior in the infant such as extrapyramidal symptoms, irritability, uncoordinated movements, and feeding problems. One case study reported withdrawal symptoms in an infant whose mother was taking fluphenazine during pregnancy; these symptoms were responsive to treatment and did not appear to affect later development[13].

Haloperidol (Haldol®): This antipsychotic medication has been in use for TS for about 4 decades. With the exception of early reports of 3 infants with limb defects, there have been no reports of structural defects in infants that can be linked with exposure to this medication. As with any medication that may affect behavior, the newborn may experience transient behavior problems, usually in feeding behavior.

Methylphenidate (Ritalin®, Concerta®, and others): These medications are used to treat ADHD. Among two case series covering 24 pregnancies during exposure to methylphendiate for clinical use, one cardiac defect was reported[14].

Olanzapine (Zyprexa®): This antipsychotic is associated with two significant side effects, obesity and type II diabetes. There is a limited enthusiasm for using olanzapine to treat tics. It does not appear to be associated with birth defects in the limited number of cases reported.

Pimozide (Orap®): Two cases have reported delivery of healthy infants to mothers with TS who took the antipsychotic pimozide during pregnancy[15,16]. Infants should be observed for the same behavioral changes as discussed with the other medications.

Quetiapine (Seroquel®): No association with birth defects has been reported for this antipsychotic medication.

Risperidone (Risperdal®): Children born to women who took this antipsychotic during pregnancy have been observed with no birth defects. Infants should be observed for behavioral changes especially the extrapyramidal symptoms of muscle spasm, tremors, irritability and posture changes.

Selective Serotonin Reuptake Inhibitors: This class of drugs was developed to treat depression, but is now also used to treat anxiety and obsessive compulsive disorder. Examples of members of this group are : citalopram (Celexa®), escitalopram (Lexapro®), fluoxetine (Prozac®), fluvoxamine (Luvox®), paroxetine (Paxil®), sertraline (Zoloft®). A withdrawal syndrome has been identified in infants whose mothers have taken one of these drugs during pregnancy, especially during the 3rd (last) trimester. Symptoms that may be seen are: irritability, increased muscle tone, jitteriness, feeding difficulties (including vomiting), tremors, agitation, breathing problems. Occasionally, these symptoms are severe enough to require admission to a special care nursery. They are transient and usually subside over the first week of life. It is important to mention that many of these reports include mothers with significant psychiatric symptoms who may also have been taking other drugs. Short term follow of the infants have not demonstrated any adverse neurodevelopment defects. Long term studies, especially through school entry, are needed.

Ziprasidone (Geodon®): One case report of a woman treated with this antipsychotic throughout pregnancy and lactation describes a healthy child with normal development through a 6-month follow-up.

Federal and Drug Administration Drug Safety Communication
In March 2011, the Food and Drug Administration issued an alert about the use of antipsychotic drugs during pregnancy. There is a potential risk to newborns for the development of abnormal muscle movements that may indicate withdrawal symptoms in the infant. The infant may exhibit feeding problems, nervousness, abnormal muscle postures, sleep difficulties and breathing problems. Examples of some of the drugs that may be associated with such symptoms are: aripiprazole, clozapine, ziprasidone, haloperidol, pimozide, risperidone, quetiapine and olanzapine[17].

MEDICATIONS DURING BREASTFEEDING
Breastfeeding is the best nutrition for the infant. Mothers are often concerned about the transfer of medication and chemicals through their milk. Fortunately, the reports of adverse effects on infants from the passage of such compounds are very small. The medications that were discussed above for the management of tics, ADHD, anxiety and Obsessive Compulsive Disorder work by acting on the chemical messengers (neurotransmitters) in the brain. To date, these drugs can be found in breast milk, although in very small amounts. The few case reports have described very young infants (less than 1 month of age) with changes in behavior (feeding problems, irritability, and colic). It must be remembered that these medications act on the brain chemical messengers and the receptors on which these medications act are maturing in the infants. Even though the amount transferred is very small, it is not currently possible to predict what long term changes may occur in the neurodevelopment of the infant. The decision on when to resume medication (if it has been stopped during pregnancy) should be made after careful discussion with the mother's physician. Information on possible effects of maternal drugs during breastfeeding may be found at the LactMed data Base of the National Library of Medicine.

CONCLUSION
Although reports of effects on the fetus by maternal use of drugs for TS and associated conditions are rare, it must be appreciated that treatment during pregnancy may be associated with neonatal effects. The best plan would be no medications during pregnancy. Drugs used to treat

tic disorders including TS affect the functioning of neurochemicals in the brain. Reports of adverse effects on the infant being breastfed by a mother taking any of these medications are sparse and almost always confined to the first two months of the infant's life. It is known that these drugs do appear in breast milk, but in very low concentrations. Long term studies are needed to ascertain whether there may be subtle changes in the behavior of the child including neurodevelopment when exposure during pregnancy and/or breastfeeding occurs. As always, females who are pregnant, or intend to be pregnant, should discuss the use of all medications with their doctors.

References

1. Schwabe, M.J. & Konkol, R.J. (1992) Menstrual cycle-related fluctuations of tics in Tourette syndrome. *Pediatr Neurol* **8(1)**, 43-46.

2. Stern, J.S., Orth, M. & Robertson, M.M. (2009) Gilles de la Tourette syndrome in pregnancy: a retrospective series. *Obstet Med* **2(3)**, 128-129.

3. Sener, E.B., Kocamanoglu, S., Ustun, E. & Tur, A. (2006) Anesthetic management for cesarean delivery in a woman with Gilles de la Tourette's syndrome. *Int J Obstet Anesth* **15(2)**, 163-165.

4. Koren G, Cohn T, Chitayat D, Kapur, B., Remington, G., Reid, D.M. & Zupinsky, R.B. (2002) Use of atypical antipsychotics during pregnancy and the risk of neural tube defects in infants. *Am J Psychiatry* **159(1)**, 136-137.

5. Mendhekar, D.N., Sunder, K.R. & Andrade, C. (2006) Aripiprazole use in a pregnant schizoaffective woman. *Bipolar Disord* **8(3)**, 299-300.

6. Mervak, B., Collins, J. & Valenstein, M. (2008) Case report of aripiprazole usage during pregnancy. *Arch Women's Ment Health* **11(3)**, 249-250.

7. Mendhekar, D., Sharma, J. & Srilakshmi, P. (2006) Use of Aripiprazole During Late Pregnancy in a Woman with Psychotic Illness. *Ann Pharmacother* **40(3)**, 575.

8. Alessi, N.E. & Spalding, S. (2003) Atomoxetine and Pregnancy. *J Am Acad Child Adolesc Psychiatry* **42(8)**, 883-884.

9. Fisher, J.B., Edgren, B.E., Mammel, M.C. & Coleman, J.M. (1985) Neonatal Apnea Associated With Maternal. Clonazepam Therapy: A Case Report. *Obstet Gynecol* **66(3)**, 34s-35s.

10. Lin, A.E., Peller, A.J., Westgate, M., Houde, K., Franz, A. & Holmes, L.B. (2004) Clonazepam use in pregnancy and the risk of malformations. *Birth Defects Res A: Clin Mol Teratol* **70(8)**, 534-536.

11. Briggs, G., Freeman, R. & Yaffe, S. (2011) *Drugs in Pregnancy and Lactation.* 9th ed. Lippincott Williams & Wilkins, MD.

12. Naeye, R.L. (1983) Maternal Use of Dextroamphetamine and Growth of the Fetus. *Pharmacology* **26(2)**, 117-120.

13. Cleary, M.F. (1977) Fluphenazine decanoate during pregnancy. *Am J Psychiatry* **134(7),** 815-816.
14. Humphreys, C., Garcia-Bournissen, F., Ito, S. & Koren, G. (2007) Exposure to attention deficit hyperactivity disorder medications during pregnancy. *Can Fam Physician* **53(7),** 1153-1155.
15. Prowler, M.L. & Kim, D.R. (2009) Perinatal akathisia: implications for pharmacokinetic changes during pregnancy. *Am J Psychiatry* **166(11),** 1296-1297.
16. Bjarnason, N.H., Rode, L. & Dalhoff, K. (2006) Fetal exposure to pimozide: a case report. *J Reprod Med* **51(5),** 443-444.
17. http://www.fda.gov/Drugs/DrugSafety/ucm243903.htm

Resources

1. Motherisk Home Line - **(416) 813-6780 http://www.motherisk. org/contact/index.php**
2. Pregnancy Riskline (Utah) – **(800) 822-2229 http://health.utah. gov/cshcn/pregnancyriskline**
3. Organization of Teratology Information Services **(OTIS) – (866) 626-6847 http://www.otispregnancy.org/otis_find_a_tis.htm**
4. Briggs GG, Freeman RK, Yaffe SJ. Drugs in Pregnancy and Lactation. 8th Edition. Lippincott Williams& Wilkins. Baltimore, MD. 2008.
5. Committee on Drugs, American Academy of Pediatrics. Use of psychoactive medication during pregnancy and possible effects on the fetus and newborn. Pediatrics 2000; 105:880-887.
6. National Library of Medicine. Bethesda Maryland. LactMed search data base **http://toxnet.nlm.nih.gov/cgi-bin/sis/ htmlgen?LACT**

CHAPTER 11

BEHAVIOR THERAPY

Matthew R. Capriotti, B.S., Flint M. Espil, M.S.,
and Douglas W. Woods, Ph.D.

INTRODUCTION

When people hear the phrase "behavior therapy," they often think of a simple treatment involving punishing people for bad behavior or giving them money or candy for good behavior. Behavior therapy is actually much more complex.

Behavior therapy comes from the idea that what we do is influenced greatly by the world around us. Various aspects of the environment (people, places, situations, activities, internal experiences) change our behavior in ways that help us adapt, and these changes in our behavior usually correspond to changes in the brain. The brain's ability to adapt or change because of its interactions with the world is called neuroplasticity. Behavior therapists understand the ability of the environment to change our brains. Based on this knowledge, behavior therapists try to identify things in the environment that can be changed and make specific changes in the environment to help the brain change in a way that makes the problem less likely to occur.

Behavior therapy is a generic term and can mean many things. Many therapists, counselors, social workers, or psychologists might tell you they do behavior therapy, but what they consider to be behavior therapy might not be the specific treatment shown to be effective in scientific research. To help you find a therapist who uses only effective behavior therapy, we use specific names for the treatments described in this chapter. When you are looking for therapists, you should ask whether or not they use these specific behavioral treatments.

WHEN CAN BEHAVIOR THERAPY BE HELPFUL?

There are different behavior therapies for different problems, including tics. Many disorders that commonly occur alongside TS can be treated with effective behavioral treatments. Often, parents will find it most effective to treat these other disorders before treating tics. In the following section, these disorders and their associated behavior therapies are briefly discussed.

Attention-Deficit/Hyperactivity Disorder (ADHD)

ADHD is characterized by a longstanding pattern of inattention, hyperactivity and/or overly impulsive behavior. Behavior therapy for ADHD teaches parents to structure their children's environments in a consistent and predictable fashion. Parents are encouraged to set routines and react to children's hyperactive or off-task behavior in a calm and consistent fashion. Parents and teachers work with therapists to restructure the environment in a way that reduces disruptive behavior. Two specific "brand names" of behavior therapy for ADHD include Barkley's Parent Training and Forehand and McMahon's model. Although stimulant medications are the most widely used and effective treatment for ADHD, scientific research also supports the use of behavior therapy.

Obsessive-Compulsive Disorder (OCD)

OCD is an anxiety disorder consisting of recurrent and unwanted thoughts, worries, images, or impulses known as obsessions. People with OCD perform compulsions (physical or mental) to get rid of anxiety created by the obsessions. The most effective type of behavior therapy for OCD is called Exposure and Response (or ritual) Prevention. In Exposure and Response (or ritual) Prevention, people learn to tolerate anxiety provoking obsessions and thereby habituate to the anxiety; let the anxiety go away on its own without doing the compulsion. Over time with repeated practice, the obsessions and anxiety decrease and patients reduce their reliance on their compulsive rituals. To learn this skill, patients are intentionally exposed to, or asked to do or think about the things that make them anxious. At the same time, therapists help patients counter their natural tendency to do the anxiety-reducing compulsions, which allows habituation to take place.

Other Anxiety Disorders

Other than OCD, two very common anxiety disorders seen among children with tics are Separation Anxiety Disorder and Generalized Anxiety Disorder. Children with Separation Anxiety Disorder typically experience extreme distress when separated from their primary caregivers (usually the mother). In Generalized Anxiety Disorder, the child expresses excessive worry about everyday experiences and activities.

Cognitive-behavioral treatments for these types of anxiety disorders involve teaching the child to come in contact with things that make them anxious, relaxation training, and role plays in which children are taught to recognize physical symptoms of anxiety and practice using skills to reduce that anxiety. A variety of techniques are also used to change anxiety-causing thoughts and teach problem solving skills. A well-researched treatment for anxiety in children is Coping Cat developed by Philip Kendall.

Depression

Major Depressive Disorder is a condition in which people feel very sad for most days, lose interest in things they usually enjoy, lose their appetite, and experience feelings of worthlessness or guilt. People with depression may have a hard time getting to work, school, or other activities. A very common behavioral therapy shown to help people with depression is called Behavioral Activation. In this therapy, behavior therapists focus on the decrease in activities that accompany depression. If people can increase the number of positive activities they engage in while decreasing the number of negative activities, this should help them get out of their depression. Therapists also work with patients to improve their social and communication skills. Two other types of therapy for depression known for their effectiveness are Cognitive Therapy and Rational Emotive Behavior Therapy. Both of these therapies teach the child/adolescent to replace their biased, negative thinking styles with more accurate thoughts.

Oppositional Behavior/Explosive Behavior

Oppositional behavior, including the two common disorders of Oppositional Defiant Disorder and Conduct Disorder, is sometimes seen in children and adolescents with tics. Children with Oppositional Defiant Disorder often lose their temper, argue, defy requests, deliberately annoy others, and are often angry or resentful. Those with Conduct Disorder show a pattern of violating the rights of others and social norms. Violent acts, aggression, destruction of property, stealing, and setting fires are all behaviors commonly seen in adolescents with Conduct Disorder. One common behavioral treatment for these disorders shown to have some effectiveness is called Parent Management Training.

Pervasive Developmental Disorders

This group of disorders consists of Autistic Disorder, Rett's Disorder, Childhood Disintegrative Disorder, Asperger Syndrome, and Pervasive Developmental Disorder Not Otherwise Specified. These disorders may involve delayed social skills, stereotyped behavior (repeated behaviors such as rocking or hand flapping), and a narrow but intense focus on certain activities. Many children with Pervasive Developmental Disorders also show a delay in language development. Behavior therapists or applied behavior analysts work with children to help identify and learn social skills, learn behaviors to improve daily functioning, and if necessary, train language skills.

WHAT IS BEHAVIOR THERAPY FOR TOURETTE SYNDROME?

Interest in behavior therapy for TS has grown in recent years, but the idea of using such treatments dates back to the early 1970s. At the time, little was known about the origin of TS. Individuals with TS were often described as having "nervous tics" or "nervous habits." Of course, we now know that tics are much more complicated than "nervous habits." Thanks to advances in biological sciences, we now know that tics are caused by a combination of genetics and certain biological processes within the brain. Although early behavior therapy for tics was called Habit Reversal Training (Habit Reversal Training was based on the prevailing notion at the time that tics were "nervous habits"), those who currently develop and use behavior therapy for TS fully acknowledge that tics are caused by biological processes and are not voluntary or bad habits. Modern-day behavior therapy for TS is based on the idea that while tics are caused by genes and biology, then can often be effectively managed through behavior therapy techniques. The most recently developed and comprehensive form of behavior therapy for TS is called Comprehensive Behavioral Intervention for Tics (CBIT).

CBIT is an individually tailored approach to the management of TS that relies on collaboration between the patient, his/her family members, and the therapist. Patients have weekly, hour-long appointments for about eight weeks.

The first 1-2 sessions of CBIT focus on teaching the patient and family about TS and behavior therapy for the problem, as well as creating a "tic-neutral environment" and deciding the order in which tics should be treated. Normally, CBIT therapists focus on treating the most bothersome tic first and work down the child's list of tics to eventually treat the least bothersome tic.

To create a tic-neutral environment, the patient and therapist first try to decide what happens in the patient's life that makes the tics more problematic than usual. This is done by doing a special type of interview called a "function-based assessment." During this interview, the therapist looks for two types of tic-worsening events. Antecedent events include things that happen before the tics occur that result in the tic getting temporarily worse. Examples of antecedents include being around certain people, having negative emotions such as stress, being tired, or participating in certain activities (e.g. watching TV, eating dinner, doing an assignment at school). In contrast, consequences are things that happen after the person tics or because the person is ticcing. Common consequences of tics include particular social reactions to the tics or being allowed to avoid something difficult when tics start to occur.

After deciding which events may be making the tic worse, the therapist works with the patient and family to change these antecedents and consequences in order to make tics happen less frequently. In addition to making subtle changes to the patient's daily environment, CBIT teaches relaxation skills because of research showing that stress and anxiety can make tics more difficult to manage.

The therapist also teaches the patient more direct tic-management skills. This part of the treatment is based on the older habit reversal training treatment. In this part of treatment, a new tic is treated during each week of therapy. For each tic, the therapist does three things: awareness training, competing response training and social support training. The first step is "awareness training", in which patients are taught to become more aware of when the tic happens and is about to happen. After coming up with a very detailed description of the tics, the patient talks with the therapist about non-tic related topics (e.g. sports, a TV shows, the weather) and signals when the tic happens during the conversation by raising a hand each time he/she tics. When the patient catches himself/herself having a tic, the therapist praises the accurate detection by saying "Good" and continuing the conversation. If the patient has a tic and does not raise his/her hand, the therapist gently states, "Remember to raise your hand," and continues the conversation. This process continues until the patient can detect all or nearly all of the times the tic occurs. The training then begins to teach patients to become more aware of the way their body feels just before they tic. Most people with TS experience some sort of sensation just before that specific tic occurs. This is called the "premonitory urge." Awareness training aims to increase patients' detection of these sensations or urges to tic.

After the patient has become aware of the tic and its preceding urge, competing response training is started. In competing response training, the patient and therapist identify a physical response or "exercise" the patient can use when he/she tics or feels the need to tic. Each tic the patient has will have a different competing response and competing responses will be harder to do for some tics than for others. As a result, your therapist may plan to spend more time in session on tics that are harder to treat.

Social support involves having people close to the patient provide encouragement and support for the practice of skills taught during therapy. Parents, siblings, spouses, or roommates often act as the main social support persons. In CBIT, this person is taught to compliment the patient for practicing the competing response exercises and gently remind the patient to practice the exercises when the support person notices the patient is ticcing and does not appear to notice and/or be practicing the competing response. It is important to emphasize that effort to manage the tics is what is being either praised or prompted. Support people are instructed never to react to how often the patient is ticcing. Reprimands or punishment for having tics have no place in behavior therapy for TS.

The therapist may choose to use a special reward system to make the child more motivated to practice his or her CBIT skills. However, just as praise is given for practicing the competing response exercises and *not* for the reduction of tics *per se*, rewards are earned for practicing competing responses and otherwise following the CBIT treatment plan, regardless of how often the tics occur.

Although the treatment sessions are where tic management skills in CBIT are taught, the most important work in CBIT occurs outside of session. The success of competing response training and function-based interventions depends in large part on the child and his/ her parents ensuring the work is done correctly. Also, CBIT involves "homework" in which both patients and parents/significant others record the frequency of the patients' tics for a short amount of time each day. These records are essential for CBIT therapists to monitor the effectiveness of treatment.

DOES BEHAVIOR THERAPY WORK?

Behavior therapy is an effective treatment for TS. Recently, the TSA Behavioral Sciences Consortium completed a large-scale randomized controlled trial (the kind of study that provides the best test of how well a therapy works) to test CBIT. The results were published in *the Journal of the American Medical Association* in 2010. In this study, 126 children and adolescents with TS were randomly selected to receive either CBIT or a control therapy known as supportive psychotherapy, in which therapists provided information about TS and discussed issues that the client may have been experiencing due to TS, but did not provide specific recommendations about how to manage tics. The study included both children who were taking medication to control their tics and those who were not.

Children in the CBIT group improved significantly more than children in the supportive psychotherapy group. Following the standard 8 sessions over 10 weeks, 53% of children receiving CBIT were rated as either "very much improved" or "much improved" by their therapist, compared to 19% in the supportive psychotherapy group. Also, the average tic symptom reduction for those receiving behavior therapy (31%) was similar to what has been found in other studies looking at medication for tics (35-36% reduction). Of those whose tics were "very much" or "much" improved, 87% continued to experience beneficial effects 6 months after treatment. This finding suggests that behavior therapy for TS is not merely a way to temporarily reduce tics, but rather an enduring treatment that teaches skills to help in the long-term management of the disorder.

CONCERNS PARENTS OFTEN HAVE ABOUT BEHAVIOR THERAPY FOR TICS

Parents of children with tics often have questions and concerns about behavior therapy for TS. Some of the more common questions are listed below:

Will Suppressing Tics Cause An Outburst Of Tics Later?

Parents sometimes wonder whether suppressing tics leads to a large, explosive outburst of tics later on. This has come to be known as a "rebound effect", or the eventual outburst of all the tics that have been suppressed throughout the day. Although this concern is quite common, many studies have shown that the rebound effect does not typically happen as a result of behavior therapy.

Will Treating One Tic Make The Others Worse?

Parents often wonder whether treating one tic will make the others worse. Research on behavior therapy for tics has shown no worsening of other, untreated tics. In fact, sometimes untreated tics even improve.

What If The Competing Response Replaces The Old Tic?

If children are learning one set of movements to replace a tic, won't the new response just become a new tic? Fortunately, behavior therapy for tics in children has not shown this to be the case. Children learn to use their competing response when needed, and as the urge to tic decreases, the need to use the competing response follows suit.

Will Doing CBIT Impair My Child's Ability To Concentrate On Other Things?

Many parents worry that using the skills from CBIT will distract their children from focusing on schoolwork and other activities that demand attention. When children with tics are asked to suppress their tics without any instruction, the ability to focus on other tasks does become slightly impaired, at least temporarily. In contrast, CBIT teaches children very specific skills to use in order to manage tics. In studies using CBIT, children do not report any decrease in their ability to focus on schoolwork and other activities that demand higher levels of attention.

Does The Availability Of CBIT Mean I Should Stop Using Medication?

Deciding whether or not to stop using medication is a decision families should *always* address with their prescribing physician. Results from the research show that behavior therapy can be effective for individuals regardless of whether or not they are taking medications for tics.

Where Can I Find A Trained Behavior Therapist?

Finding behavior therapists that are well-trained to provide CBIT can be difficult at this time. Some helpful resources for locating tic specialists are the Tourette Syndrome Association, Inc. (TSA) and the Association for Behavioral and Cognitive Therapies (ABCT) websites. The TSA website (http://www.tsa-usa.org/index.html) has a special section with information and referral information for individuals looking for help with tics. The ABCT website (http://www.abct.org/Home/?m=mHome&fa=dHome) has a "Find a Therapist" page where individuals can search for qualified therapists in their communities. Although the ABCT site does not specifically list TS among the specialties in the search criteria, searching for a therapist who specializes in OCD or Exposure Therapy might be your best option.

References

1. Azrin, N.H. & Nunn, R. G. (1973) Habit reversal: A method of eliminating nervous habits and tics. *Behav Res Ther* **11,** 619-628.

2. Conelea, C. A. & Woods, D. W. (2008) Examining the impact of tic suppression in children and adolescents with tic Tourette syndrome. *Behav Res Ther* **46,** 1193-1200.

3. Nathan, P., & Gorman, J. M. (Eds.) (2007). A guide to treatments that work (3rd ed.). Oxford, NY.

4. Piacentini, J., Woods, D.W., Scahill, L., Wilhelm, S., Peterson, A.L., Chang, S., Ginsburg, G.S., Deckersbach, T., Dziura, J., Levi-Pearl, S. & Walkup, J.T. (2010) Behavior therapy for children with Tourette disorder: A randomized control trial. *JAMA* **303,** 1929-1937.

5. Verdellen, C.W.J., Keijsers, G.P.J, Cath, D.C., & Hoogduin, C.A.L. (2004) Exposure with response prevention versus habit reversal in Tourette's syndrome: A controlled study. *Behav Res Ther* **42,** 501-511.

6. Woods, D.W., Miltenberger, R.G. & Lumley, V.A. (1996) Sequential application of major habit-reversal components to treat motor tics in children. *J Appl Behav Anal* **29,** 483-493.

7. Woods, A. W., Piacentini, J. C. & Walkup, J. T. (Eds.). (2007) Treating Tourette syndrome and tic disorders: A guide for practitioners. Guilford, NY.

8. Woods, D. W., Piacentini, J. C., Chang, S. W., Deckersbach, T., Ginsburg, G. S., Peterson, A. L., Scahill, L.D., Walkup, J. T. & Wilhelm, S. (2008) Managing Tourette syndrome: A behavioral intervention for children and adults. Oxford, NY.

CHAPTER 12

DEEP BRAIN STIMULATION FOR TOURETTE SYNDROME

Michael S. Okun, M.D., Herbert Ward, M.D., Irene Malaty, M.D.,
Nikki Ricciuti, RN, CCRC, LMHC, Candy Hill, Ph.D.,
and Kelly D. Foote, M.D.

INTRODUCTION

Deep brain stimulation (DBS) is a promising treatment option for TS patients. However, the surgery is reserved for patients whose motor and/or vocal tics significantly impact the quality of life despite maximal doses of multiple medications. The media buzz surrounding DBS for TS has been exciting; however, it has created many questions for patients and their families to consider. In this chapter, we provide a brief overview of DBS and discuss how this approach might be used as a treatment for TS. We also address many of the questions that have been asked about this approach as treatment.

DEEP BRAIN STIMULATION

DBS is a relatively new procedure that utilizes an implantable electrode which may be used in place of, or in conjunction with ablative brain procedures such as pallidotomy or thalamotomy (where a portion of the brain is irreversibly destroyed by burning it). Patients with Parkinson disease, tremor, dystonia, or obsessive compulsive disorder (OCD) who are medically refractory to therapy, and who have no cognitive (thinking) difficulties or "minimal" cognitive dysfunction may be appropriate candidates. There are also other expanding indications such as depression, cluster headache, epilepsy, and now TS.

The procedure is U.S. Food and Drug Administration (FDA) approved for Parkinson's disease, essential tremor, dystonia and OCD. The currently available technology is manufactured by the Medtronic corporation, although many companies are now involved in the development of brain hardware. The DBS lead has four electrode contacts (quadrapolar), and depending on the disorder and/or the brain target, one may use variably sized contacts with different spacing arrangements. Each contact can be activated utilizing monopolar (the current when passed to the brain is shaped like a big globe or sphere) or bipolar stimulation (the current when passed to the brain is shaped like an oval), and multiple settings can be adjusted for individual patient needs. The settings that can be adjusted may include the pulse width (how big each pulse of stimulation is), frequency (how many times per second we give each pulse), and amplitude of stimulation (how much voltage we pass through the lead). The DBS electrode is implanted into a specific area within the brain, and is attached to a programmable pulse generator. The pulse generator, or neurostimulator, is implanted in a subcutaneous pocket below the clavicle and connected to the DBS electrode in the brain via a tunneled extension cable that passes subcutaneously (under the skin) over the clavicle and across the posterior aspect of the neck and skull (the pulse generator is just like a cardiac pacemaker except the wire goes to the brain).

Figures 1 & 2 are pictorial representation of the DBS device that displays the DBS lead which is inserted into the brain with the connector wire and neurostimulator (battery).

WHY WOULD DBS HELP TO AMELIORATE TS?

DBS has the potential to "neuromodulate" abnormal signals that occur deep within the brains of patients with TS. So far, researchers have probed into several areas in the brain of people with TS (the centromedian thalamus, the internal globus pallidus, the external globus pallidus, and the anterior limb of the internal capsule), and they have had mixed success. The best target for "neuromodulation" or for changing the signals has yet to be determined; however, it is clear that in some patients the introduction of electrical stimulation has very positive effects.

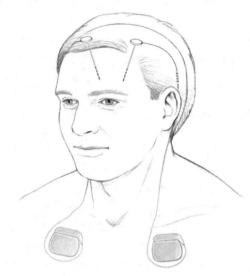

Figure 1. Frontal View of DBS Device

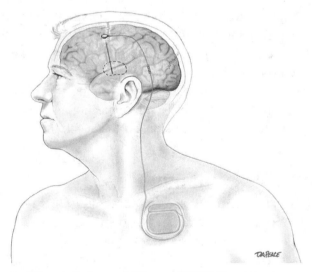

Figure 2. Lateral View of DBS Device

MULTIDISCIPLINARY/INTERDISCIPLINARY SCREENING PRIOR TO DBS AND WHY IT IS IMPORTANT

An important concept to understand when evaluating any potential DBS candidate is that successful surgery usually requires a multi/ interdisciplinary approach. The general neurologist or general practitioner can serve an important role in identifying and in triaging potential DBS candidates; once triaged, a potential candidate should be evaluated comprehensively by an experienced team. The team should optimally include a psychiatrist who is experienced in evaluating movement disorders, a neurologist who is experienced in movement disorders scale administration, a stereotactic trained neurosurgeon, and a neuropsychologist. In some cases, a social worker, and a physical, occupational, and speech therapist may be useful. Additionally, adequate imaging must be performed (usually a Magnetic Resonance Imaging and/or Computed Tomography), and the results of each part of the screening should be discussed in a DBS meeting/board. These meetings/boards are usually similar in format to medical oncology boards where members are charged with deciding on the best comprehensive tumor therapy approach for both the patient and the family. The group should meet, exchange findings, and then stratify the risk: benefit ratio for each patient. The multi/interdisciplinary group should be aware of, and address the list of symptoms a patient "expects" will improve with surgery. The results of this team meeting should be shared with the patient and the family to be sure expectations may be reasonably addressed by the overall decision on the recommended approach to therapy.

CANDIDATES FOR DBS

Probably the most crucial step for successful DBS is careful patient selection. Careful consideration of patient characteristics will directly impact outcome. Despite the widespread use of DBS, there are no standardized criteria for selection of candidates. Generally, the most suitable candidates have little medical comorbidity (other diseases besides TS), few if any cognitive deficits, and a stable psychiatric status. DBS is a powerful treatment for motor and vocal tics, but it is has not to date proven effective for non-motor symptoms such as obsessive compulsive traits, attention deficit, and other behavioral disorders. The Tourette Syndrome Association has recently published recommendations for surgery in the *Journal of Movement Disorders*. Below are some general considerations for patients and families.

1. The diagnosis of TS must be made by an expert psychiatrist and/or a neurologist.
2. The Yale Global Tic Severity Scale should be performed and must reveal incapacitation with severe distress, self-injurious behavior, and/or quality of life disruption. OCD, Depression, and Attention Deficit Hyperactivity Disorder are not exclusionary provided tics are the major difficulty requiring surgical intervention.
3. Age must be >25 by FDA guidelines and Tourette Syndrome Association Inc. guidelines and many studies may exclude TS patients younger than this age. Age is a relative contraindication only as there may be exceptional cases where younger patients may require a surgical intervention.
4. The patient's TS symptoms must be medication refractory and have failed conventional medical therapy for tics. To meet the medication refractory criteria, subjects must have been treated by a psychiatrist or neurologist experienced in TS (usually treated with at least three different pharmacological classes: an alpha-adrenergic agonist, dopamine antagonists (typical and atypical), and a benzodiazepine). In some cases tetrabenazine is another medication that may be useful for treatment of Tourette syndrome.
5. Patients must have received stable and optimized treatment of comorbid or other medical, neurological, and psychiatric disorders for the previous 6 months.
6. If the patient has a tic that is focal or addressable by botulinum toxin treatment this should be considered.
7. Patients must have treated and stabilized psychiatric disorders if present: anxiety, depression, bipolar disorder or other psychiatric disorder.
8. Patients must be screened for dementia or cognitive dysfunction that will place the patient at risk for worsening cognition (thinking), and/or may impact the ability to cooperate with tasks involved in the study.
9. Patients should be aware there is a behavioral tic intervention available called Comprehensive Behavioral Intervention for Tics.

COMMITMENT IS REQUIRED FOR DBS THERAPY

DBS requires a significant time commitment, and patients and families must be motivated to undergo not only the procedure but also the challenges associated with the pre-operative workup and the significant follow-up after the procedure. The family must be willing to return for multiple evaluations and they must realize that the average patient may be programmed 4-8 times in the first six months following surgery. Most experienced centers have begun to shy away from performing DBS in patients unless there is a spouse or a committed caregiver (especially a caregiver that can provide travel). Many patients and families are under the erroneous impression that DBS therapy is a "light switch," and once it is turned on the journey comes to an abrupt and miraculous end. The truth is, following activation of the device, there are still many battles to be endured with both DBS programming (there are thousands of potential settings), and medication changes. Patients and families must be willing to agree to multiple programming and to medication adjustments. Patients can ultimately become DBS failures simply from a lack of commitment to the process.

RESULTS OF DBS FOR TOURETTE SYNDROME

The largest open label, uncontrolled and unblinded study of TS DBS utilized a single brain target and was published in a recent issue of the *Journal of Neurology, Neurosurgery & Psychiatry*. Although three targets have been tested in small series for TS, the authors of the aforementioned work focused on the centromedian thalamus-parafascicular complex (inclusive of the ventralis oralis). The globus pallidus interna and externa, and the anterior limb of the internal capsule/nucleus accumbens have also emerged as potentially effective areas for amelioration of medication refractory tic; however, they have been less studied. Servello and colleagues reported in the largest series to date that in 18 patients, DBS significantly decreased motor tics, but the therapy was less effective for phonic tics. The therapy was said to not be as "promising" as the authors had hoped in addressing behavioral manifestations of TS, despite improvements on the social scale of the Yale Global Tic Rating Instrument. Many groups are experimenting with other targets and approaches to TS, and to date there is no consensus except that motor tic responds better than behavioral manifestations of the syndrome.

COMPLICATIONS ASSOCIATED WITH DBS

DBS has many short and long term "potential" complications. Despite these problems, the vast majority of well-selected patients rate their experience with DBS as overwhelmingly positive. The DBS device does not have a blood supply, so infection is a potential problem and can occur in 5% or more of cases. Further, the microelectrodes and/ or the DBS lead could injure a blood vessel, causing bleeding or alternatively a stroke that may lead to weakness, numbness, changes in vision, and/or changes in speech. The DBS device might also fracture/ break, migrate out of position, or malfunction. DBS often affects the speech, and particularly verbal fluency (getting words out of the mouth of patients). There can be worsening of cognition or mood, and in rare cases associated suicidal thoughts (another reason why patients must be carefully screened and followed). The addition of a second DBS lead in the opposite side of the brain may also increase the risk for walking, talking and thinking problems.

The largest risk of a DBS procedure is failure to achieve the patient's pre-operative expectations, and this is why it is absolutely critical that both patients and physicians have focused pre-operative discussions.

WHAT IS A DBS FAILURE, AND HOW CAN I AVOID BECOMING A DBS FAILURE?

As studies of DBS for TS proceed, we must be mindful of potential failures. For example, failures in triage or sending the right patients for surgery; failures in screening with a complete multidisciplinary team; failures in performing the procedure carefully; failures in programming the device properly; and failures in post-operative medication management are possible and we must make all attempts to avoid these pitfalls. A DBS failure can also result from inadequate pre-operative expectations or a failure of the DBS team to properly educate the patient pre-operatively as to what to "reasonably" expect. Since DBS is relatively new for TS, it is reasonable to believe that some patients undergoing the procedure will not benefit significantly and research will help us in differentiating the right candidates and the right brain targets as we forge forward.

CONCLUSION

What is needed for DBS to move forward as a viable therapy for medication refractory TS are prospective, blinded, randomized, follow-up studies of the promising brain targets. We must keep both an open mind, as well as rigorous control of all the factors that may influence results including target, current technology, inclusion/exclusion criteria, age at entry into a study, a true definition of medication refractoriness, stimulation parameters, location of the active lead contact, and exploration into motor, non-motor, and quality of life issues. These studies should be undertaken by experienced multidisciplinary teams, and should be guided by clinical trials. Evaluations should be performed by blinded raters. Despite the positive results of this and other studies, we must learn the lessons which have resulted in DBS failures in other disorders, and make serious early attempts to avoid them in TS. Currently we are aware of two centers that have received FDA investigational device exemptions to perform Tourette DBS studies in the United States (Case Western, Cleveland OH, and University of Florida, Gainesville—also with a National Institutes of Health funded study). There may be other centers with FDA and/or institutional review board clearance to perform DBS, and as we become aware of these centers we will post them to the website.

References

1. Zabek, M., Sobstyl, M., Koziara, H. & Dzierzecki, S. (2008) Deep brain stimulation of the right nucleus accumbens in a patient with Tourette syndrome. Case report. *Neurol Neurochir Pol* **42(6),** 554-559.
2. Albert, J.M., Maddux, B.N., Riley, D.E. & Maciunas, R.J. (2009) Modeling video tic counts in a crossover trial of deep brain stimulation for Tourette syndrome. *Contemp Clin Trials* **30(2),** 141-149.
3. Neuner, I., Podoll, K., Janouschek, H., Michel, T.M., Sheldrick, A.J. & Schneider, F. (2008) From psychosurgery to neuromodulation: Deep brain stimulation for intractable Tourette syndrome.*World J Biol Psychiatry* 1-11.
4. Dehning, S., Mehrkens, J.H., Muller, N., & Botzel, K. (2008) Therapy-refractory Tourette syndrome: beneficial outcome with globus pallidus internus deep brain stimulation. *Mov Disord* **23(9),** 1300-1302.
5. Okun, M.S., Fernandez, H.H., Foote, K.D., Murphy, T.K. & Goodman, W.K. (2008) Avoiding deep brain stimulation failures in Tourette syndrome. *J Neurol Neurosurg Psychiatry* **79(2),** 111-112.
6. Shields, D.C., Cheng, M.L., Flaherty, A.W., Gale, J.T. & Eskandar, E.N. (2008) Microelectrode-guided deep brain stimulation for Tourette syndrome: within-subject comparison of different stimulation sites. *Stereotact Funct Neurosurg* **86(2),** 87-91.
7. Maciunas, R.J., Maddux, B.N., Riley, D.E., Whitney, C.M., Schoenberg, M.R., Ogrocki, P.J., Albert, J.M., & Gould, D.J. Prospective randomized double-blind trial of bilateral thalamic deep brain stimulation in adults with Tourette syndrome. *J Neurosurg* **107(5),** 1004-1014.
8. Servello, D., Porta, M., Sassi, M., Brambilla, A. & Robertson, M.M. (2008) Deep brain stimulation in 18 patients with severe Gilles de la Tourette syndrome refractory to treatment: the surgery and stimulation. *J Neurol Neurosurg Psychiatry* **79(2),** 136-142.
9. Riley, D.E., Whitney, C.M., Maddux, B.N., Schoenberg, M.S., & Maciunas, R.J. (2007) Patient selection and assessment

recommendations for deep brain stimulation in Tourette syndrome. *Mov Disord* **22(9)**, 1366; author reply 1367-1368.

10. Poysky, J. & Jimenez-Shahed, J. (2007) Patient selection and assessment recommendations for deep brain stimulation in Tourette syndrome. *Mov Disord* **22(9)**, 1366-1367; author reply 1367-1368.

11. Kuhn, J., Lenartz, D., Mai, J.K., Huff, W., Lee, S.H., Koulousakis, A., Klosterkoetter, J. & Sturm, V. (2007) Deep brain stimulation of the nucleus accumbens and the internal capsule in therapeutically refractory Tourette-syndrome. *J Neurol* **254(7)**, 963-965.

12. Shahed, J., Poysky, J., Kenney, C., Simpson, R., & Jankovic, J. (2007) GPi deep brain stimulation for Tourette syndrome improves tics and psychiatric comorbidities. *Neurology* **68(2)**, 159-160.

13. Mink, J.W., Walkup, J., Frey, K.A., Como, P., Cath, D., Delong, M.R., Erenberg, G., Jankovic, J., Juncos, J., Leckman, J.F., swerdlow, N., Visser-Vandewalle, V., Vitek, J.L. & Tourette Syndrome Association, Inc. (2006) Patient selection and assessment recommendations for deep brain stimulation in Tourette syndrome. *Mov Disord* **21(11)**, 1831-1838.

14. Flaherty, A.W., Williams, Z.M., Amirnovin, R., Kasper, E., Rauch, S.L., Cosgrove, G.R. & Eskandar, E.N. (2005) Deep brain stimulation of the anterior internal capsule for the treatment of Tourette syndrome: technical case report. *Neurosurgery* **57(4Suppl)**, E403; discussion E403.

CARNEGIE PUBLIC LIBRARY
202 N Animas St
Trinidad, CO 81082-2643
(719) 846-6841

CHAPTER 13

COMPLEMENTARY AND ALTERNATIVE THERAPIES

Katie Kompoliti, M.D.

INTRODUCTION

There is a growing interest among patients in complementary and alternative medicine (CAM). CAM refers to a wide range of therapies outside the domain of mainstream Western medicine that are used for the purpose of disease prevention, amelioration of symptoms, or health promotion in general. Conventional medicine is medicine as practiced by medical doctors, doctors of osteopathy and by allied health professionals, such as physical therapists, psychologists, and registered nurses. Complementary medicine is used in conjunction with conventional medicine; for example, massage and acupuncture may be used in addition to pain medications to help decrease pain. Alternative medicine is used in place of conventional medicine; for example, using herbs rather than antidepressant medications to treat depression. The boundaries between CAM and conventional medicine are not absolute, and specific CAM practices may, over time, become widely accepted and therefore part of the conventional medical system.

People choose alternative treatments for many different reasons. These reasons may include the desire to have more control over one's own healthcare decisions, or the hope of finding treatments that work better or have fewer side-effects than traditional healthcare treatments. Since more and more people are using the Internet as a source of medical information, this trend has grown enormously. People now have access to information not only from traditional sources, but also from individuals who share their personal experiences using alternative treatments. Unfortunately, as with all information on the Internet, there is no way to verify the accuracy or usefulness of such information. Another frequent reason for trying CAM is it is more in line with one's own values, worldview, spiritual or religious philosophy, or beliefs regarding the nature and meaning of health and illness. For these people, such holistic philosophies concerning health make the use of CAM more attractive than current, traditional treatment. Others may believe that current medical practices are too impersonal, too technologically oriented, too complex or too costly. The 2007 National Health Interview Survey, which included a comprehensive survey of CAM use by Americans, showed that approximately 38 percent of adults use CAM. Additionally, 11.8% of children aged 17 years and under are reported users of some form of CAM. The majority of users choose to add to (complement) their traditional treatments. Typically, patients do not discuss the use of alternative treatments with their doctor(s).

The purpose of this chapter is to discuss what is known and unknown about such treatments to help people make informed decisions about the CAM treatments used in TS. Examples of some of these treatments will be discussed in detail.

ORIGINS AND USE OF CAM

Before the modern era of medicine, healers made medicines from natural sources, especially plants and animals. In some societies today, such practices are still the main forms of treatment. In the 19th and 20th centuries, scientists began to study these medicines to understand how they work. Using modern techniques to understand the chemistry and biology of these treatments, scientists learned to make and improve the natural remedies. When substances were found to be helpful in treating illness, they were produced as medicines. In our discussion here, we will call treatments that have been studied and refined by medical scientists as "traditional".

Most medicines, whether traditional or alternative, relieve only the *symptoms* produced by illness in most cases. Rarely do they cure the disease itself. An example of a treatment that cures illness is antibiotics that kill the bacteria that cause infections. Another example is chemotherapy that cures some forms of cancer. Chronic illnesses such as diabetes, heart failure, arthritis, and asthma can be helped by treatment, but the underlying illnesses are still there. This means that symptoms can recur when the treatment is stopped. Even though treatments can help relieve the symptoms of many neurological disorders including Tourette syndrome, scientists do not know the cause of TS, and a cure has not been found. We know that chemicals in the brain called neurotransmitters play a role in TS. However, we do not know how these neurotransmitters work, nor do we understand very well which parts of the brain are involved in producing the disorder.

The Tourette Syndrome Association. Inc. (TSA) is working with scientists, physicians, advocacy groups, families and others to help build better understanding about what causes TS. With this information, newer and better treatments can be studied. The TSA supports healthcare practices that emphasize safety and effectiveness. No treatment, whether traditional or alternative, is fully "safe" or fully "effective". It is the policy of the TSA to stand behind and support solid scientific research that studies the safety and effectiveness of treatments. Unfortunately, many treatments (and especially CAM treatments) have not been well studied, so reliable information about safety and effectiveness is limited. Traditional medicines can be prescribed and used only after many years of research have proven them to be safe and effective. Since CAM treatments are not regulated by the Food and Drug Administration (FDA), information about their safety and effectiveness is not controlled. It is important to understand that this does not mean that a CAM treatment is unsafe or will not work. Instead, this means that the information is not yet available to prove that it does work or that it is safe.

In the following sections, we will discuss several CAM treatments and will share, when available, what is known about the safety and effectiveness of these treatments. According to the National Center for Complementary and Alternative Medicine, CAM treatments can be divided into 5 categories:

- Biologically based therapies, Nutritional therapies
- Mind-body medicine
- Manipulative and body-based practices
- Energy therapies
- Alternative medical systems

BIOLOGICALLY BASED THERAPIES, NUTRITIONAL THERAPIES

Biologically based therapies or nutritional therapies include dietary supplements, herbs, vitamins, and minerals. Many substances in this category have been promoted to reduce motor and vocal tics, as well as the associated conditions that might accompany Tourette syndrome including attention deficit hyperactivity disorder (ADHD), obsessive compulsive disorder, oppositional defiant disorder, and anger outbursts.

In 1994, Congress passed the Dietary Supplement Health and Education Act, which removed supplements from the same degree of scrutiny by the Food and Drug Administration (FDA) that is required for traditional medicines. The manufacturers do not have to prove to the FDA the safety and efficacy of supplements before they are marketed. Rather, it is up to the FDA to demonstrate that a dietary supplement or an herb is unsafe once it is already in the market.

The consumer has to consider the possibility that what's on the label may not be what's in the bottle. Analyses of dietary supplements sometimes find differences between labeled and actual ingredients. In a recent survey of 40 popular herbal dietary supplements, the Government Accountability Office, found trace amounts of at least one potentially hazardous contaminant in 37 of the products tested. Some preparations have been found to contain heavy metals (lead, mercury, and arsenic), bacteria, environmental chemicals and drugs (caffeine, corticosteroids, benzodiazepines such as Valium® and diuretics).

There has been no clear scientific demonstration of what is the actual active ingredient or ingredients in any herb and some herbs contain dozens of potentially pharmacologically active compounds. Many herbs and pharmaceutical drugs are therapeutic at one dose and toxic at another. Interactions between herbs and drugs may increase or decrease the beneficial or toxicological effects of either component. Many herbs will interact in a negative way with prescription drugs when both are taken together, and some may change how a drug is metabolized by the body. For example, in transplant patients, self-medication with St John's wort has led to a drop in plasma levels of the immunosuppressant drug cyclosporine, causing transplant rejection in some patients[1].

When deciding to start a supplement, one has to keep in mind that although many dietary supplements (and some prescription drugs) come from natural sources, "natural" does not always mean "safe." For example, the herbs comfrey and kava can cause serious harm to the liver. It is therefore important to look for reliable sources of information on dietary supplements. Patients should seek reliable, evidence-based information about the safety and efficacy of specific therapies and therapists.

DIETARY SUPPLEMENTS

Herbals

Ningdong granule, a traditional Chinese medicine compound composed of eight different Chinese herbs has been tested in several clinical trials, one of them against placebo in a blinded fashion and was found to be superior to placebo in TS. Side effects included loss of appetite and constipation. Larger scale studies and reproducibility of these results are required[2].

There is a body of research indicating that supplementation with Pycnogenol and omega-3 fatty acids might assist symptoms of ADHD. However, rigorously designed clinical trials are missing. A study examining the effects of omega-3 fatty acids compared to placebo on tics and obsessive compulsive disorder compared to placebo in children and adolescents with TS has not been completed yet. Flaxseed oil is a rich source of the omega-3 fatty acid called alpha-linolenic acid. Flaxseed oil also has a large amount of a "lignan", a fiber-associated nutrient. Use of this compound has been shown to lower total cholesterol. Grapeseed extract and Pycnogenol® contain (among other substances) a group of chemicals called proanthocyanidins. These compounds may have a role in preventing free radical formation in the body and thus decrease the harmful effects from oxidative stress. Potential health benefits may include more rapid recovery from injury (e.g. heart attacks, stroke) and combating cancer. Many foods contain these compounds including fruits, cereals, beans, nuts, spices, chocolate and grapes. No research is available on their effects on tics and the other manifestations of TS.

Hyoscyamus and chamomilla, two homeopathic ingredients felt to decrease spasms and lessen stress respectively, have been used to address tics, albeit without systematic documentation of their effectiveness or side effects and drug interactions.

Vitamins

Generally, people living in the United States do not suffer from vitamin or mineral deficiencies unless they have a specific illness or are adhering to an unusually restrictive diet (especially what is called a "vegan" diet). It has been claimed by some that taking various combinations of vitamins will help alleviate a wide range of symptoms, including tics. Sometimes, the dose of vitamins recommended is many times higher than is normally thought necessary for good health (megavitamin therapy). Large doses of some vitamins such as A and D, E and K can accumulate in the body and cause toxicity.

One vitamin that has been implicated in the pathogenesis of TS is B6. Some authors have postulated that the central event in the etiology of Tourette syndrome is magnesium deficiency. Magnesium is required for the tissue uptake of the vitamin B6, consequently magnesium deficiency can prevent the body from utilizing B6, thus producing a functional B6 deficiency. B6 deficiency on the other hand causes increased magnesium excretion leading to a further negative magnesium balance[3]. An open label study has evaluated the effect of combined magnesium and B6 administration for tics with encouraging results, prompting the investigators to design a randomized placebo-controlled study to confirm these preliminary findings.

Probiotics

Probiotics are live microorganisms (in most cases, bacteria) that are similar to beneficial microorganisms found in the human gut. They are also called "friendly bacteria" or "good bacteria." Probiotics are available to consumers mainly in the form of dietary supplements and foods. There is no research on probiotic use and TS symptom control.

Special Diets

Many behavioral symptoms in children have been blamed on what is in their diet, and the claim of a connection between sugar intake and ADHD has been especially prominent. These views have led to claims that increased sugar, lack of certain fatty acids, or exposure to other food substances may cause a "food allergy", resulting in behavioral symptoms. Food allergy is a term that may include true allergy to a component of a food or a direct effect on the gastrointestinal tract that does not require a true allergic pathway (food intolerance). Elimination diets can resolve symptoms of true allergy or intolerance and have been suggested as a treatment for the symptoms of TS.

The effect of refined sugar and food additives on ADHD patients is controversial, with some, but not most studies showing that sugar and food additives can worsen ADHD symptoms. A review of 16 studies with ADHD children found that sugar challenges were associated with worsened symptoms of inattention and hyperactivity in 4 studies, little change in 11 studies, and improvement in ADHD symptoms in 1 study. Diets free of food coloring, natural salicylates, and food preservatives, such as benzoate, nitrates, and monosodium glutamate have been widely used to treat children with ADHD, although the studies have been inconsistent[4].

Heavy Metals

It is sometimes thought that either an excess or a deficiency of certain heavy metals may play a central role in causing tics. One study that assessed serum copper levels in patients with TS found that some of them had low serum copper levels. The significance of this is still uncertain. Because of similarities in the clinical presentation of magnesium deficiency and tics, it has been proposed that magnesium deficiency may cause tics and studies assessing the effect of administration of magnesium and B6 for the treatment of tics are underway (already outlined in more detail in the vitamins section). Other heavy metals that are used in supplement cocktails by TS patients are zinc and iron, although there are no research studies supporting the use of any of them. It is interesting that not only a lack of minerals has been associated with causing tics, excess has been linked to tics as well. Mercury intoxication has been reported to have caused tics in a case report of a Chinese boy.

Hair analysis is a test in which a sample of a person's hair is sent to a laboratory for measurement of its mineral content. This analysis has been used to evaluate a person's general state of nutrition and health or to detect predisposition to disease. The results of hair analysis have been used as the basis for prescribing supplements or performing chelation therapy (see below). Biological specimens such as hair are frequently subject to contamination (chemicals used for cosmetic purposes, environmental exposures, etc.) or can vary based on hair color, length, age, gender and numerous other factors. No correlation has been established between hair and tissue levels of trace elements. Finally, most commercial laboratories have not standardized their results, and no normal ranges have been defined. For these reasons, most physicians do not believe that hair analysis of trace elements is a valid test for identifying body excesses or deficiencies, nor a valid basis for prescribing treatment.

Chelation
Chelation therapy was developed during the 1950s as a way to cleanse the blood and blood vessel walls of toxins and minerals. Although chelation therapy plays a role in the treatment of lead or other heavy metal toxicity, there is limited scientific evidence about safety or effectiveness for any other conditions. Additionally, chelation may cause many adverse effects or, rarely, even death.

MIND-BODY MEDICINE
Mind-body medicine focuses on bi-directional interactions between the brain ("mind") and the body. The brain and body are viewed as two pieces of a single system, rather than as two separate systems. The health of one piece directly shapes the health of the other. In mind-body medicine, the influences of the brain include one's emotions, behavior, perceptions, and spirituality.

The National Center for Complementary and Alternative Medicine (NCCAM) lists a wide range of interventions in the mind-body medicine category. These interventions include relaxation, hypnosis, guided or visual imagery, meditation, yoga, biofeedback, tai chi, qi gong, cognitive-behavioral therapies, group support, autogenic training, spirituality, mental healing, and prayer.

Self-healing, rather than physician-healing, is an important part of mind-body medicine approaches, in part because of the identity of "mind", and therefore of "self", as being effective toward well-being. Some of the mind-body medicine approaches are familiar and established in the practice of Western medicine, e.g., cognitive-behavioral therapies in the treatment and prevention of depression or anxiety and group support used widely in healthcare. Other methods are so commonly used that "self-care", rather than professional-based or CAM interventions seems to be the best description for these activities. For example, within the past year, more than one-third of all American adults have used self-prayer directed to a health concern.

Another popular approach in the management of TS symptoms (and in many other chronic illnesses) is peer support groups. There is a general assumption that there is value in sharing one's experiences with others who have similar experiences. Among the perceived benefits to peer support is an increase in self-awareness and, therefore, in personal control.

Each of the mind-body medicine approaches must be considered individually with regard to safety and efficacy; therefore, it is not reasonable to cluster all approaches together as one and the same. A lot of mind-body medicine approaches are considered safe and are often affordable or cost-free. As with many CAM approaches, mind-body medicine approaches can offer the appeal of self-empowerment.

Still, mind-body medicine approaches are not totally without risk. Because of the emphasis on "self", a mind-body medicine approach that does not produce significant results may be interpreted as a failure in oneself, rather than as a failure in the approach itself. One therefore risks feelings of fault, guilt or abandonment. Also, there are risks inherent in pursuing an unproven approach as an alternative to (rather than as a complement of) a proven approach. In addition, the efficacy of many mind-body medicine approaches are considered not to be measurable, as each individual is unique. When an assumption is made that the efficacy of an approach is non-measurable, neither patients nor therapies can be compared or tested by standard scientific research methods.

Biofeedback
Biofeedback is a specialized type of training that allows people to gain control over their body's reactions that are ordinarily unconscious and automatic. It involves the use of electronic equipment to monitor specific, often unconscious body reactions and feedback the information to the person. Depending on the body function targeted, electrodes or other sensors are applied on various parts of the body. These electrodes or sensors are connected to a computer that provides instant feedback about the body function that is targeted for control. Electroencephalograms are tests that record brain wave activity. Electroencehalograms biofeedback is based on the concept that brain wave activity can be

altered voluntarily after the information about the changes in their own brain wave activity is "fed back" to the person. This treatment has been used to improve tics, compulsions and ADHD.

Hypnotherapy

Hypnosis brings about a state of mind where a person's normal critical or skeptical nature is bypassed, thus allowing for acceptance of suggestions. This state of heightened receptivity for suggestions (induction) is developed with the cooperation of the individual. It is followed by the therapeutic intervention which consists of providing positive suggestions. Participants in hypnotherapy are usually taught to discriminate their tics from other movements. Simultaneously, self-hypnosis training is started, using relaxation techniques and visual imagery for deepening of the trance. Improvement is sought by instructing the subjects to bring the relaxed feelings back with them when the session is over. A recent study reported positive effects of self-hypnosis training on 33 children and adolescents. More supportive evidence is still required, since this study assessed efficacy based on self-report of improvement and did not assess long term effect of self-hypnosis[5].

MANIPULATIVE AND BODY-BASED PRACTICES

Manual therapies include a variety of CAM approaches that emphasize "manipulation" (using hands) and body-based therapies. Approaches include massage therapy, chiropractic manipulation, reflexology and acupuncture. More than half of all visits to CAM practitioners are for manual therapies. The basis for these therapies emphasizes the health of body structures and systems, including bones, joints, muscles, blood, lymphatics and others, and typically assumes that the body is self-regulating with the ability to repair itself. Manual therapies are practiced as preventive health measures, to promote general well-being, and for the treatment of a wide range of conditions

Massage Therapies

Massage can help the symptoms of TS through alleviating muscular pain that may cause tics or to relieve pain that results from having tics. Also, massage may help people relax and reduce stress—both states that may help to reduce tics. Potential risks are rare.

Chiropractic Therapy

Chiropractic manipulations primarily use spinal manipulation to relieve a wide range of symptoms. Chiropractic therapy is sought by patients with TS to relieve pain resulting from the tics. Potential risks include discomfort in the area of the body that is being treated, as well as more serious risks including stroke, paralysis, and damage to the bones and nerves of the spine. There is no research addressing the effects of chiropractic manipulations on tics or their consequences.

Acupuncture

Acupuncture is a widely used treatment option that aims to promote the flow of negative energy. During the procedure, needles are inserted beneath the skin at special points on the body, and mechanical or electrical stimulation is applied to the needles. Some research has shown that acupuncture helps reduce nausea in cancer, dental pain and other illnesses. Acupuncture is generally considered to be safe. Infection, including hepatitis, is a potential risk. There is a publication in the *Journal of Traditional Chinese Medicine* reporting favorable effects of acupuncture on TS, but better designed studies are necessary to confirm such effect[6].

Reflexology

Reflexology is based on the principle that congestion or tension in any part of the foot mirrors congestion or tension in a corresponding part of the body. These parts, known as reflex points can also be found on the hands and other body parts; however, the most commonly treated area is the feet. Reflexology has been used to address many conditions, including pain and stress. There are only anecdotal reports on favorable effects of this technique on the manifestations of TS but no systematic report of case series or study.

ENERGY THERAPIES

Energy medicine includes a broad array of CAM approaches, and addresses forms of energy which can be measured, such as static magnetic and electromagnetic forces, and energies which cannot be measured, such as a vital energy of life. Energy therapies include magnet therapy, healing touch, light therapy and reiki. The basis for energy therapy stems from the belief that an illness results from energy disturbances.

Magnet Therapy

Magnets have been used for health purposes for centuries. Currently, magnets are widely marketed for pain control. Preliminary scientific studies of magnets for pain have produced mixed results. Overall, there is no convincing scientific evidence to support claims that magnets can relieve pain of any type. Some studies, including a recent National Institutes of Health clinical trial for back pain, suggest the possibility of a small benefit from using magnets for pain. However, the majority of rigorous studies have found no effect on pain. There are only isolated testimonial cases reporting efficacy of magnet therapy in TS but no scientific research investigating their efficacy.

Reiki

Reiki is a self-healing practice originating from Japan, used to promote overall health and well-being, as well as relief from specific disease-related symptoms and side effects of conventional medications. Reiki practitioners place their hands lightly on or just above the person receiving treatment, with the goal of facilitating the person's own healing response. Reiki has not been studied scientifically for any medical condition including TS.

ALTERNATIVE MEDICAL SYSTEMS

Homeopathy

Homeopathy is based on the assumption that the body's ability to cure itself can be stimulated by highly diluted substances. There are two main principles of homeopathy. The principle of similar (or "like cures like") states that a disease can be cured by a substance that produces similar symptoms in healthy people. The principle of dilutions (or "law of minimum dose") states that the *lower* the dose of the medication, the *greater* its effectiveness. According to the 2007 National Health Interview Survey, an estimated 3.9 million U.S. adults and approximately 900,000 children used homeopathy in the previous year. Two of the three randomized, controlled trials of homeopathy, for attention deficit hyperactive disorder reported results in favor of homeopathy although the primary outcome measure was the Connor's Parent Symptom Questionnaire, thus relying upon parent self-report, a potential source of bias[7].

Naturopathy

Naturopathy is based on the theory that "impurities" cause disease, so the body works to purify itself. Naturopathic practitioners view their role as supporting the body's inherent ability to maintain and restore health, and prefer to use treatment approaches they consider to be the most natural and least invasive. On a practical level, they employ many different treatment modalities, such as nutrition counseling, including dietary changes (such as eating more whole and un-processed foods), use of vitamins, minerals, and other supplements, herbal medicines, homeopathy, hydrotherapy, physical medicine, such as therapeutic massage and joint manipulation, exercise therapy, and lifestyle counseling. There is no evidence supporting naturopathy as a treatment for TS symptoms.

Ecology

Clinical ecology is based on the belief that some people have immune system weaknesses that increase their sensitivity to low levels of substances in the environment that otherwise cause no problem for most people. Predisposing risk factors are thought to include infection due to a fungus (*candida*), a deficient or inadequate diet, and/or food intolerance. Symptoms may involve every organ of the body, but central nervous system and behavioral symptoms seem to predominate. Avoidance of the substances presumed to cause the problem is a major goal of this therapy. Additionally, diluted extracts of the suspected substance given under the tongue or injected under the skin are used to diagnose or treat the person's symptoms. There is no evidence for using this approach in managing TS.

Aromatherapy

Aromatherapy states that pleasant odors may promote relaxation, and this may enhance self-healing by the body. These odors come from "essential" plant oils, seeds, flowers, and roots. The oils can be rubbed on the skin or put into a special drink. Various aromas from these oils can be quite pleasant and have been said to improve one's sense of well-being. There is no scientifically sound evidence for treating TS with this approach.

CONCLUSION

The use of complementary and alternative therapies is appealing to many in the TS community for various and important reasons. The TSA continues to encourage interested practitioners to do the needed research that will study the safety and effectiveness of CAM treatments in TS. To date, these treatments have rarely been studied in a scientific way.

Although often viewed as "natural" and "harmless", the TSA recommends that consumers remember a number of facts before considering the use of such therapies. While generally safe, CAM therapies are not regulated by the FDA, so that the level of safety and effectiveness has not been proven. A product is not necessarily harmless, even if it is natural. Many natural products contain contaminants, impurities, or a large number of different active ingredients. Some of these may interact and interfere with prescription medications. CAM therapies can also have side effects, just as is true for traditional medications.

It has long been known that the symptoms of TS will wax and wane in intensity and frequency. When symptoms improve, therefore, it is often difficult to be certain whether the improvement was due to treatment (whether traditional or alternative) or due to the natural fluctuations seen in the disorder.

A report of success in one person is no guarantee that the same therapy will help someone else. This unpredictability creates a dilemma for physicians as well as patients. While some of the alternative treatments may be effective, there is no objective way for the physician or the consumer to sort through and choose one over the other.

Physicians should seek continued and updated knowledge about therapeutic options available to their patients, whether they are main stream or CAM. The first guideline for the use of any intervention should be to seek reliable, evidence-based information about its safety and effectiveness. More than anything, when considering a therapeutic decision, both the doctor and the patient should apply common sense to balancing risks and benefits. If the therapy is both safe and effective, then the decision is easy. Thus, the level of evidence required for evaluating efficacy can be small when there is little to no risk of harm from the therapy, especially when other therapies have failed. Likewise, the level of evidence for efficacy required to endorse a particular CAM therapy would be quite high when that therapy is risky and safer, more effective treatments are available. Factors to be included in a risk/benefit analysis when considering CAM therapies include the individual's personal beliefs, cultural values and practices, and therapeutic goals. The desire to "try everything" is a strong one, but caution must be used. The use of CAM therapies requires the same careful decision making processes as does the decision to use prescription medications. In all things, "caveat emptor"—buyer beware—is useful advice[8].

References

1. Fugh-Berman, A. (2000) Herb-drug interactions. *Lancet* **355,** 134-138.
2. Zhao, L., Li, A.Y., Lv, H., Liu, F.Y. & Qi, F.H. (2010) Traditional Chinese medicine Ningdong granule: the beneficial effects in Tourette's disorder. *J Int Med Res* **38,** 169-175.
3. Grimaldi, B.L. (2002) The central role of magnesium deficiency in Tourette's syndrome: causal relationships between magnesium deficiency, altered biochemical pathways and symptoms relating to Tourette's syndrome and several reported comorbid conditions. *Med Hypotheses* **58,** 47-60.
4. Curtis, L.T. & Patel, K. (2008) Nutritional and environmental approaches to preventing and treating autism and attention deficit hyperactivity disorder (ADHD): a review. *J Altern Complement Med* **14,** 79-85.
5. Lazarus, J.E. & Klein, S.K. Nonpharmacological treatment of tics in Tourette syndrome adding videotape training to self-hypnosis. *J Dev Behav Pediatr* **31,** 498-504.
6. Wu, L., Li, H. & Kang, L. (1996) 156 cases of Gilles de la Tourette's syndrome treated by acupuncture. *J Tradit Chin Med* **16,** 211-213.
7. Hunt, K. & Ernst, E. (2011) The evidence-base for complementary medicine in children: a critical overview of systematic reviews. *Arch Dis Child* **96(8),** 769-76.
8. Kemper, K.J., Vohra, S. & Walls, R. (2008) The use of complementary and alternative medicine in pediatrics. *Pediatrics* **122,** 1374-1386.

Resources

1. Complementary and Alternative Medicine Use Among Adults and Children: United States, 2007. National Health Statistics reports, CDC and National Center for Health Statistics.
2. Herbal Dietary Supplements: Examples of Deceptive or Questionable Marketing Practices and Potentially Dangerous Advice. United States Government Accountability Office, Testimony before the Special Committee on Aging, US Senate.

Websites

http://nccam.nih.gov
www.healthwatcher.net
www.imconsortium.org

CHAPTER 14

THE PSYCHOSOCIAL ASPECTS OF TOURETTE SYNDROME: A FAMILY GUIDE AND PERSPECTIVE

Mary May Robertson, M.B. Ch.B., M.D., D.Sc. (Med), D.P.M., F.R.C.P., F.R.C.P.CH., F.R.C.Psych.

INTRODUCTION

This Chapter provides some background on the "psychosocial aspects" of TS. Intriguingly, even though TS has been known since the descriptions by Dr. Itard of the Marquise de Dampierre in 1825, and by Dr. Georges Gilles de la Tourette in 1885 (see Chapter 17), little has been formally studied in this area. Maybe this is because TS was thought to be rare for a long time, and so numbers of patients with TS in clinics were relatively few (when compared to those with asthma or epilepsy) and so initial studies on TS were clinical descriptions (e.g. describing what tics and their characteristics were), (see Chapter 2). Subsequently, studies looked at TS and how it changed over the person's lifetime, and then studies followed on the psychiatric conditions associated with TS (see Chapter 3), how common TS is worldwide (see Chapter 5), the genetics and other possible causal factors (see Chapters 7 & 8) and treatment (see Chapters 9,10,11&12). For a brief outline of the psychosocial consequences of TS see Table 1.

DEFINITION OF PSYCHOSOCIAL AND ITS RAMIFICATIONS IN PEOPLE WITH TS

What does the term psychosocial mean? Well, the *Oxford English Dictionary* defines the word psyche as "mind, spirit, soul", and we know that disorders dealing with the mind are "psychiatric" or "psychological", and doctors and some professionals who treat people with these difficulties are "psychiatrists" and "psychologists". Social is essentially defined as "living with others (i.e., specifically not living a solitary life) and within a society". I would also add the actual physical environment to the "psychosocial world"—for all inhabitants, and particularly for those with TS.

Psychosocial is often bandied around as a word, but pragmatic and useful definitions are surprisingly difficult to come by. According to *Wikipedia,* "psychosocial" refers to one's psychological development in, and interaction with, a social environment. Of importance is that the individual may not necessarily be fully aware of this relationship with his/her environment.

Any person affects her/his social (i.e., other people) and physical environments, and also vice versa, and so it is, with a person with TS. This will hopefully be demonstrated in this chapter. In the case of the individual with TS, there are numerous ways in which the individual reacts and interacts with the environment, and some of these aspects will be described. The individual lives within a family, attends school and hopefully higher education follows; they may also have a family (partner and/or children) of their own. All these individuals live within society at large which is influenced by many factors, including the media which comprises newspapers, magazines, television and an ever enlarging Internet and social networking sites; the media now has enormous influence on opinions of people in many countries.

As will be seen, individuals with TS may be frankly excluded from society. The tics *per se* may alter the individuals interaction with the environment, the co-morbid disorders (specific psychiatric disorders), especially Attention Deficit Hyperactivity Disorder (ADHD), may also adversely affect a person's lifestyle, as the individual's quality of life may suffer and his or her parents or caregiver's life may be unduly burdened. Prior to diagnosis, parents of youngsters with TS may blame themselves for their child's symptoms and this may not be helped by health professionals, suggesting that symptoms are a result of bad parenting. The individual with TS may become depressed, have school phobia, stigma, and, in addition, may have to live with the possible side effects of medications used to treat the symptoms. Education or lack thereof and employment, or again, lack thereof will certainly affect the individual with TS, and there may be a circular spiralling of matters (e.g., tics and ADHD that may lead to exclusion, poor education, lack of employment and drug and alcohol abuse).

BACKGROUND OF THE DEMOGRAPHICS OF TS
A good way to introduce the subject is to acknowledge that TS:

- is a common disorder that affects up to 1% of the population
- occurs in all social classes
- individuals have an average IQ on intelligence tests
- affects males 3-4 times more than females.

Importantly, most people with TS in the community are probably undiagnosed and have mild TS, and you, the reader, may know someone with mild TS who is undiagnosed. It is fair to suggest that the person with mild TS and no other psychiatric disorders probably has very few, if any, psychosocial difficulties (as a result of TS).

THE HISTORY OF TS ILLUSTRATING PSYCHOSOCIAL CONSEQUENCES OF HAVING TS
The best way to begin a chapter such as this is with reference to the history of the disorder. Both Dr. Itard in 1825 and Dr. Gilles de la Tourette in 1885 wrote about a French noblewoman, the Marquis de Dampierre, who is a very good example of the psychosocial effects of TS on the individual and also society. The Marquis began to have movements as a child; she then made loud noises; and finally, she had coprolalia (swearing). She was of noble status, and the latter symptom was unacceptable within her society. She was forced to live as a recluse until she died—so that she would not be heard to swear and would not bother anyone. Thus, she lived a socially-isolated, lonely life ostracised by society with all the psychosocial sequelae it entailed.

ON BEING A PERSON WITH TS AND SOME OF THE PSYCHOSOCIAL ISSUES

A good section with which to next illustrate the subject of psychosocial issues in people with TS may well be the stories of people with a diagnosis of TS, as well as the stories of some successful people with TS; that is, those who overcame many psychosocial difficulties. However, relatively few individuals with TS have documented their personal experiences. Dr. Zinner, a physician in the USA (see Chapter 15), and Dr. Hollenbeck, a neuroscientist (see Foreword), have clearly described living with TS, but a few more will be mentioned, as each individual with TS is special and may bring slightly different insights into having the disorder. For those readers truly interested in TS, it is recommended that they read the rest of the original stories, as the present authors admit to only hinting at their experiences, not really doing them justice.

Joseph Bliss in 1980 wrote the first fairly ground-breaking personal account about "living with and documenting living with TS" from 8-67 years old, when he highlighted the *inner sensory experiences* or impulses of TS, which precede, accompany and follow the motor and vocal/phonic tics. He also emphasized how bodily sites become sensitised, and how the movements are *intentional* acts aimed at satisfying and eliminating unfulfilled sensations and urges. He also highlights how sensory impressions ("phantom sensations") may be projected onto other persons, objects or even imagined objects. He even tells us how these barely perceptible emergent sensations can be recognised and controlled through substitution or extinction (a prophetic precursor to the basis of several behavioral therapies). He finally "confesses" how coping with these sensations and their consequences and current affairs and *LIFE,* on the other hand, creates an almost "dual citizenship" within the person. Mr. Bliss' first memory of having tics was as a young boy at the age of 8 in 1918, when his loud vocalisations in school brought mortifying criticism from his teacher. His next encounter was with a prominent psychiatrist in 1947 who told Mr Bliss that "nothing could be done for him" and that he "should save his money and spend it on the education of his children"; he was devastated and left in despair. In 1976, he was overwhelmed by "sensory impulses dancing around his head, eyes, ears neck. He notices, to his wonder, that he can direct the impulse sensations from one site to another, almost at will, by simply shifting his attention" . . . "Fascinated he does it again and again", admitting that he has "been stalking this thing for over 35 years with a single minded determination to find something that would give [him—me] a clue, a direction, to the meaning of the problem. Only in 1978 was he given a diagnosis of TS by Dr. Arthur K. Shapiro in Scarsdale, New York, one of the physician pioneers of TS.

Peter Hollenbeck, Ph.D., a prominent Neuroscience Professor and past Co-Chair of the TSA Scientific Advisory Board also gave a moving and erudite account of living with TS. Dr. Hollenbeck recalls how, only three weeks and "five orange pills" after his TS diagnosis (in his late 30s), he was "awash in an entirely novel internal tranquillity" for the first time in his life; only then did he realize how his whole life, decades to date, had been dominated by "an incessant internal drumbeat . . . of background noise . . . background hum . . . sensation, distraction, complex impulses"—and only then he realized that other people did not hear his internal drumbeat! He shares with us that the sensory experiences of his "constant [TS] companion" and their "complex, challenging and enigmatic *internal* world is the obvious core of TS, the birthplace of tics"—distal to the basal ganglia but proximal to the tics—and the real target of treatment. He goes on to describe other people with TS and the "wounds inflicted on them" [by being tormented by other people about their TS]. He describes TS as "a disorder of the onlooker" rather than that of the patient/person with TS. He himself was mocked and teased by neighbours, classmates and even teachers. Dr. Hollenbeck attributes much of his "success" as a person (as opposed to a successful academic) to his supportive family and home environment, where he was always made to feel "normal".

Dr. Lance Turtle in the UK summarizes his degrees, curriculum vitae and "life status" as "BSc, MBBS, MRCP, Ph.D., DTMH, Gilles de la Tourette Syndrome" and is the only practicing physician and only non-American to have documented his personal TS story. He was born in 1973 to middle class professional parents and lived in London, UK. His early life was unremarkable; he developed normally and he began to tic at the age of 4. Dr. Turtle remembers having first being singled out [because of his *undiagnosed* TS] at the age of around 10 years when his choirmaster at school suggested to his parents that he be put on "tranquillizers" as with his marked head tic, he may "look very odd to our audiences". At high school he was bullied because of his loud vocal tics and felt he was a "misfit" as other youngsters called him "twat", threatening him and swearing at him to "shut up" whilst the pupils were trying to go to sleep at night in the communal dormitory. His tics also affected his family, and when he was 15 to 17 years, the whole family went to a counsellor—which did not help the tics, but did help the family cope (1988-1990 in UK). He clearly recalls sensory experiences which began at about 14 years and has persisted into adulthood. He described university and medical school as a great success, with a waning of tics, making many good friends, increasing in self-confidence, excellent grades [present author's note], and it was only during a lecture at medical school that he was diagnosed by the present author (MMR). He graduated with MBBS (M.D. in USA), Ph.D. and went on to specialise in infectious disease, and the last time MMR saw him was in 2010 when he delivered a lecture to an international audience; it was excellent. In his paper, Dr. Turtle clearly describes his subsequent analysis of the sensory experiences and may well astound readers as he states that tics are actually *voluntary (in response to an "irrepressible physical urge")*; he describes his premonitory sensations as a "welling up in the centre of his head, moving upward and then seeming to fly out of the top". Also, he clearly distinguishes these from conventional sensory stimuli, suggesting they lay "somewhere between somatic sensation and imagination". He ends on a moving philosophical note, noting that as a successful physician, he has cultivated the slightly eccentric persona that TS has made him and that although he would rather not tic—he is comfortable with them and would not consider being "formally diagnosed" [in a consultation], nor take any of the new treatments; TS is part of him and has found his label and his place in life.

Jim Eisenreich, the USA Major League Baseball player, was interviewed by Fuerst in 1999. He obtained his diagnosis at the age of 23 years, even though he knew that "he was different" from the age of six. At 23, he was prescribed haloperidol and for the first time in his life he felt that he had less tics and that he was normal, calmer, with more self-control, increased self-confidence and self-esteem.

What all three individuals highlighted as a "core" symptom of their TS were the premonitory or internal subjective sensations; these sensations (premonitory urges, sensory tics, sensory phenomena, sensory experiences, "just-right" perceptions, "not-just-right" phenomena and "incompleteness") are very important parts in TS and also the tic-related Obsessive Compulsive Disorder (OCD) subtype.

Few of the successful and articulate individuals discussed above and in Table 2 (especially those who documented their own experiences) had coprolalia; most had late or no formal diagnoses, and they described the internal sensory experiences as the core of the "TS internal world" that no other person [without TS] can *really fully understand*. It is this internal sensory world that we must all try to always understand—to even try and grasp some of the psychosocial consequences of having TS.

It is possibly worth considering whether these individuals succeeded despite *or* because of having TS. My personal view is that they would have succeeded anyway—and it is unlikely that it is *because of* TS. As the main etiology/cause of TS is considered genetic, were it because of TS (i.e., TS is an advantage), one would expect TS to be an advantage for all and lead to increased survival and prevalence—neither of which are the case.

PERSONAL ANECDOTES AS A DOCTOR WHO HAS SPECIALISED IN TS: EXPERIENCES IN THE PUBLIC DOMAIN

It may also be appropriate to document in this chapter some experiences of being a doctor specialising in TS, and interacting with individuals with TS *outside* the TS clinic. In other words, as members of the general public may do—albeit less informed.

I have served as a medical advisor to several television documentaries on TS, and as a fore-runner to one, I collaborated with the TV crew making a short film. A patient from our clinic very kindly volunteered to help with the making of the film. We decided to take a lunch break and went to a local restaurant. Being in the TS clinic as a doctor, one is used to hearing coprolalia (swearing), seeing copropraxia (rude gestures), as well as a host of other TS symptoms, such as spitting. However, to sit next to someone (the same person) at lunch in an ordinary restaurant was different, as I could see, at first hand, how the symptoms of swearing, rude gestures and spitting could affect the individual with TS and also those with them in the public domain.

A well-known neurologist and his TS-patient-friend visited me in my office. My resident, who had never met a person with TS, entered the room, and the person with TS grabbed my colleagues' genitals (a tic); my colleague was very non-plussed. The four of us then went to a local pub, and I can still hear the person with TS saying, "Don't make a fuss, don't make a fuss"; was he being prophetic? We ordered our drinks and, as we were enjoying a drink and chat, he suddenly had a huge arm tic and knocked the glass of beer out of my hand; our group was suddenly the centre of attention. I immediately began to go to the bar to explain, but the man with TS went instead and won the heart of the publican and the crowd; despite his awkward tic—he was an ambassador for TS.

There is a well-known delightful European man with TS who "has to" touch females' earrings. I well remember the first time it happened to me at a conference—and, realising it was a tic or his Obsessive Compulsive Behavior (OCB), it did not bother me at all, but it was interesting to watch the reactions of women who were less acquainted with his particular TS-behavior!

I am a keen opera fan, and once, at an opera, sat in front of a person with TS. I am prepared to say that it was unlikely that he was *diagnosed* with TS as he was mild, but he had numerous symptoms, three of which were frequent throat clearing, coughing, and sniffing (some of the most common phonic/vocal tics). Although I was sympathetic as a doctor—it was *not* good to have the arias and poignant moments interrupted by continuous noises. For me this brought up a huge "conflict of interest" situation—of course he should have been there, also enjoying the opera. However, if I had a head cold or flu with coughing and sniffing, I certainly would *not* have attended the performance.

Finally, I used to be a final medical degree (MBBS, MBChB [UK]; M.D. [USA, Europe]) examiner. My patients with TS were very good "examination subjects" as they were pleasant, cooperative, reliable, and would arrive at the examinations in good time, could give a good history and had obvious symptoms (tics) from which lively discussion with the candidate could be had. One TS patient of mine came into the examination room, and even before I could introduce him to my "very-proper-pin-striped-suited-male-Professor" colleague, the patient kissed me (Non-obscure Socially Inappropriate Behaviors) and put his 3rd finger in the air (copropraxia), asking very nicely how I was and saying how happy he was to be of assistance to us and the students. My colleague was very non-plussed; it was just as well that he himself was not being examined!

As can be seen from the anecdotes, for me to experience and observe the effect of the symptoms of TS *in the public domain*, demonstrated to me just how very difficult life can be not only for the person with TS at times, but also for members of the public.

THE TYPES OF TS AND THE PERSON WITH TS LIVING IN THE SOCIAL WORLD

It is important to realise that the individual with TS who has to interact with society and vice versa, is first and foremost a person, a whole person who just happens to have tics, some with tics only, whilst the majority (up to 90%) also have co-morbid disorders, which has been demonstrated in both clinics and also in the community settings. The most common co-morbid disorders are ADHD, obsessive compulsive behaviors (OCB) and disorder (OCD), depression, oppositional defiant disorder, conduct disorder (CD), autistic spectrum disorders and personality disorders (see Chapter 3).

Nevertheless, the individual also has the needs of any person. S/he has to live, eat, sleep, develop, be educated, obtain a job, have friends, love and be loved and maybe marry and have children. Some of the symptoms of TS, including the tics and the co-morbid disorders, may interfere with several of these ambitions.

It is now recognised that there is more than one TS type, despite the fact that all main diagnostic criteria have both always suggested, and indeed stipulated, that TS is a unitary condition. Recent studies have challenged this notion. Much of the evidence for TS not being a unitary condition comes from studies employing complicated statistical analyses, all of which demonstrated that TS is not a single condition, with many types being reported. However, in all studies that have examined this issue specifically, one factor has included simple motor and phonic/vocal tics. So, it seems important to say again, that the individual with TS is first and foremost a whole person; a whole person who may just happen to have simple tics only (about 10%), while many (up to 90%) also have other disorders (outlined in Chapter 3); so, there are many "Faces" of the person with TS. Psychosocial difficulties may occur because of the tics, the co-morbid disorders or often moderate to severe TS, which includes *both* severe tics and the co-morbid disorders.

PSYCHOSOCIAL ASPECTS OF THE ACTUAL TICS AND, IN SOME CASES, UNUSUAL TICS ON THE INDIVIDUAL WITH TS

It may seem obvious that loud or continuous noises (vocal tics) and severe motor tics will have psychosocial consequences. The severe or unusual tics may result in the person with TS having to keep away from other people, being excluded from a class at school or asked to leave a theatre performance; all of these situations would clearly have a negative effect on the person with TS, such as depression and/or having a lower Quality of Life (QOL).

Coprolalia (the swearing tic) occurs in approximately 20%-30% of TS people in clinics but in few members in the community with TS. The TSA suggests that an overall figure for coprolalia in TS is 10% (that is it is uncommon). However, clearly the shouting of obscenities in public has adverse effects on the individual with coprolalia and also members of the public.

Spitting as a tic occurs in several patients with TS and once again, spitting in the presence of others, especially at meal times causes the person with TS enormous distress, but is also awkward for the people who are in their company.

Very obvious tics such as severe arm flailing are documented; although, it is unclear how common they are. These patients could be viewed as "aggressive" whereas they mean no harm to others—and this would have obvious consequences on the patient and those around them.

Pain is a prominent feature of TS that is mostly due to the discomfort produced by sudden or extreme ticcing, including severe neck tics, and tics that cause fractures and nerve damage. This pain can be treated by pain killers at times, but in the author's clinic, more than one patient had to wear a neck collar to prevent any further physical injury and pain. Clearly wearing a neck collar, in addition to the tics, further highlights the individual as "being different" from others.

Some people with TS (about 6% of males and 4% of females in TS clinics worldwide) have had "sexually inappropriate behaviors", including masturbating in public, a male exposing his genitals, indecent assaults on children of the opposite sex and transvestitism. Clearly these affect the person with TS (e.g., resulting in legal action) and members of the public (being shocked).

THE RELATIONSHIPS BETWEEN PSYCHOSOCIAL FUNCTIONING AND SCHOOLING IN YOUNG PEOPLE WITH TS

Over a dozen research studies have now looked at the effects of TS and especially the association with ADHD in children. Other studies have examined different aspects of youngsters with TS and psychosocial issues, and a few studies have specifically examined the schooling of youngsters with TS.

Studies comparing people with TS-only and TS+ADHD have shown, in general, that those with TS-only are similar to healthy youngsters, whilst those with TS+ADHD have lower performance IQ's, school problems, poor peer relationships, disruptive behaviors, more depression and anxiety and poorer social adaptation than children with TS-only or healthy children. In addition, one study showed that the parents' "parenting style" (the way the parents treated and interacted with their child) affected the child's psychosocial outcome.

While discussing schooling and youngsters with TS, it may be worth mentioning that school phobia (also known as separation anxiety disorder) has been documented in youngsters with TS as a side effect of several antipsychotic medications, especially haloperidol and pimozide. The symptom may disappear on discontinuation of the drug or treatment with tricyclic antidepressants, which are often given for depression or OCD (see Chapter 9).

So, in conclusion, it appears that in general it is the ADHD which occurs in about 60% of TS patients that affects individuals with TS adversely rather than the pure tics *per se*. In addition, psychosocial factors, such as parenting style, may influence the psychopathology in TS; however, some of the medications that doctors prescribe for the tics may have psychosocial consequences as well.

PSYCHOSOCIAL STRESS *PER SE* IN YOUNG PEOPLE WITH TS

There have been few studies which have examined or invoked a role of psychosocial stress in the prediction of severity and thus prognosis of TS. The first was a case study over one and a half years which did show that stressful life events produced an increase in tics, and symptom levels varied markedly according to the boy's activity.

Only one group (Dr. Leckman's at Yale) has examined this formally and showed that psychosocial stress is a factor which makes tics worse at the time of the stress, that TS subjects experienced more stress than a control healthy group of youngsters, and that psychosocial stress is predictive of future depressive symptoms. Current levels of psychosocial stress and depression were moreover independent predictors of future tic severity. They did another study looking at streptococcal infections (see Chapter 8) and showed that the streptococcal infections were predictive of increased tics and OCD severity, and more importantly, the infections, increased by a factor of three, the power of psychosocial stress in predicting future tic and OCD severity.

What can be said, therefore, is that psychosocial stress does make tics worse at the time of the stress and in the future and that, if people with TS also have a streptococcal infection, this will increase the effect of the stress threefold.

CULTURE (SOCIAL ENVIRONMENT) AND PSYCHOSOCIAL FUNCTIONING IN YOUNG PEOPLE WITH TS

Culture, TS and psychosocial functioning has only been studied once, by the present author and her colleague. They compared young people with TS in the United Arab Emirates with similar patients in London, UK. The amounts of OCD and ADHD were similar. There was more coprolalia in the UK and it was associated with TS severity. Co-morbid oppositional defiant disorder and CD were also higher in the UK, but this was not linked to any other clinical feature or severity of TS. This raises the issue of the social environment (culture) and other influences on the behavior of these young people. It was suggested by us that other possible reasons for increased behavioral problems in the UK compared to the UAE may be due to socio-cultural-religious differences between the two countries (for example, in the UAE family stability is high, with both parents present, often large supportive families, with a strongly embedded religious discipline, a strong patriarchal presence, and more strictly enforced moral and legal codes). This may demonstrate another effect on psychosocial functioning in youngsters with TS, namely culture.

THE EFFECTS OF TS ON PSYCHOSOCIAL FUNCTIONING IN ADULTHOOD

When examining psychosocial functioning of adults with TS, one may question how youngsters with TS function at school (and attain grades), obtain employment, enter and graduate from tertiary education, have successful careers and successful long term friends, and eventually long term partners, marriages and children. Relatively few studies have, however, examined these aspects of TS.

Surprisingly, few studies have reported on adults with TS as far as psychosocial functioning. In general TS+ADHD patients have more depression, anxiety, obsessive-compulsive behaviors, and maladaptive behaviors (significantly more drug and alcohol abuse, aggression, forensic encounters) than patients with TS-only. Also, adults with TS (compared to healthy people) had poorer social adaptation and more behavioral problems than healthy people. In addition, adults with TS had higher rates of ADHD, major depression, learning disorders, and conduct disorder. In the TS individuals, measures of tic, ADHD, and OCD symptom severity correlated with worse psychosocial outcomes.

My conclusions from the studies are that clinically ascertained children with TS typically have impaired functioning as older adolescents in several psychosocial areas and high rates of co-morbid disorders. In addition, more severe tic, ADHD, and OCD symptoms in childhood are associated with poorer outcomes in late adolescence. When examined in adult TS patients, psychopathology and maladaptive behaviors seem to be associated with TS+ADHD rather than TS *per se.*

THE EFFECTS OF THE ACTUAL PHYSICAL ENVIRONMENT ON INDIVIDUALS WITH TS

Once again, few studies have examined this in detail; although, many of our patients tell us that they cannot tolerate, for example, tight shirt collars, sleeves or cuffs. A few studies have confirmed these anecdotal reports and shown the effects of heat on TS (increasing tic severity) and emotional stimuli on tic severity (again tic severity changed with emotions). Thus, it seems that indeed the actual physical environment may affect tics, whether in the mother's womb or in the person's actual physical environment.

Several studies have shown that both pre and perinatal events, including psychosocial stress, can affect not only tic severity, but also co-morbidity (Chapters 3, 7 & 14). In brief, these events (especially maternal smoking and psychosocial stress) seem to make the child vulnerable to TS more likely to show symptoms (i.e., be affected) of increased tic severity, and that maternal smoking is associated with a subsequent diagnosis of TS+ADHD in the offspring.

THE LENGTH OF TIME FROM ONSET TO DIAGNOSIS

It is a matter of concern that there is often a lag between age at onset of TS and age at diagnosis. This can have several consequences, including the parents blaming themselves for the child's behavior or problem, or the professionals accusing the parents of bad parenting. Both of these situations clearly will have adverse psychosocial consequences on the whole family.

In the medical literature, early studies showed a "diagnostic lag" of some 14 years, whereas in studies published 12 years later, only a few patients were not diagnosed until adulthood. This almost certainly is a reflection of both public and professional knowledge about TS, largely due to the efforts of the TSA in the various countries world-wide.

EFFECT OF TS ON THE PERSON AND THUS THE QUALITY OF LIFE IN PEOPLE WITH TS AND PARENTING STRESS IN TS

Many studies have relatively recently emerged documenting the QOL of individuals with TS. As may be anticipated, an individual with severe tics, in addition to added co-morbid disorders, may be expected to have significant alterations in their lives. However, this has not been much studied and only relatively recently been investigated formally, employing various, although different QOL scales. The studies' results were remarkably consistent showing that TS patients have a reduced QOL when compared with healthy individuals than general population samples, but better QOL than patients with bad epilepsy. The majority of studies, despite studying both young people and adults with TS, showed that the areas of life which contribute to this lower QOL included pain and/or physical discomfort, interference with the individuals' usual activities, poor mobility, difficulties with self-care, lack of employment, increasing age, tic severity, as well as OCB, OCD, anxiety, depression, and ADHD.

There have been far fewer studies in the area of the amounts of stress on parents and its influencing factors, in caring for children with TS. All studies reported that the stress for caring with a child with TS is high. Reasons for this increased stress included child care difficulties. Associations were also noted between parenting stress and child gender, age, school situation, parental age, family income and TS severity. More social support, not surprisingly, seems to lessen parental stress. Parenting stress was also worse for parents of individuals with TS than for parents of youngsters with, for example, a serious physical disease such as asthma. In addition, parents of youngsters with TS had more stress and seemed to develop more psychiatric disorders than parents with children with asthma. Thus, having a child with TS, particularly if TS is severe and little support is given to parents, seems to increase parental stress. It is not difficult to see why dedicated clinics staffed by experts in TS and the TSA are important in giving not only medical advice, but also providing a social support network for families that have a child or children with TS.

NON-OBSCENE SOCIALLY INAPPROPRIATE BEHAVIORS (NOSI) IN TS

NOSI is commonly encountered in people with TS, but has not been frequently studied. The most common type of NOSI includes insulting others. NOSI is usually directed at a family member or familiar person. Approximately one third of patients had resultant social difficulties and NOSI is associated with ADHD and CD, suggesting the possibility of NOSI being an impulse control disorder. It does not take much imagination to understand what effect an individual with TS and NOSI might have on others. I recall a patient living in an area with a predominantly Afro-Caribbean population, and he just shouted out the "N*   * *" word, despite the fact that some of his friends belonged to that particular population. It reached such a climax that the patient had to be re-housed out of the area on medical grounds. Another patient of mine who was in fact of Pakistani origin, would loudly shout out "Paki Paki" which is considered to be offensive, and received much criticism from his own cultural group. What is important is that neither of these patients approved of any racial slurs, but as so often happens with TS patients, these words just "burst out", so to speak.

SELF-INJURIOUS BEHAVIORS, DELIBERATE SELF-HARM (DSH), TS AND PSYCHOSOCIAL FUNCTIONING

As with NOSI, self-injurious behaviors (SIB) pose another problem to the individual with TS, and are a typical and characteristic behavior, encountered in between 14% and 60% of TS patients. This is a substantial proportion of TS individuals, whether they are in the clinic or the community. Studies have suggested that TS patients of mild/moderate severity with SIB are significantly obsessional, with OCB (e.g., presence of aggressive obsessions, violent or aggressive compulsions, and the presence of OCD). Severe SIB, on the other hand, may be correlated with variables related to affect (e.g., being depressed) or impulse dysregulation, in particular, with the presence of episodic rages and risk taking behaviors (Chapter 4).

Of practical importance with the SIB encountered in TS is that these are deliberate acts, but the intention of the individual is *neither to die* nor to actually harm themselves (e.g., in contrast to wrist cutting). Those with TS just "have to punch their face, press their eye or bang their heads." This is in broad contrast to deliberate self-harm (DSH), suicide attempts and actual suicide—which occur in people with typically different psychopathologies, such as those with personality disorders, severe major depressive illness, or psychosis which are encountered in general psychiatric practice.

In contrast, probably the worst psychosocial "outcome" of a disorder is that an individual is so distressed by the disorder and its consequences that they commit suicide. Thankfully, however, documented suicide and DSH are relatively rare outcomes for patients with TS, but should always be considered if there are symptoms of depression and/or a reduced quality of life.

RAGE ATTACKS OR EXPLOSIVE OUTBURSTS OF AGGRESSION IN TS

Rage attacks have been described in about 23%-40% of TS patients (Chapter 4). These are worrying symptoms and behaviors for family members, friends and indeed the patient with TS. These are usually sudden, explosive episodes of rage which occur in a significant number of children in TS clinics and cause considerable psychosocial morbidity. Research has not been widely documented, but it appears that most patients with "TS-rage attacks" also have other co-morbid disorders, especially ADHD and OCD, whilst some have additional oppositional defiant disorder and CD. Of note is that in general the "rage" is independent of tic severity and age of the patient. Interestingly, the rages occur in response to a mild stimulus and are often accompanied by remorse. The symptom can be difficult to treat successfully and invariably results in family and peer difficulties.

OTHER PSYCHOSOCIAL CONSEQUENCES ASSOCIATED WITH HAVING TS

Although psychiatric disorder occurs in up to 90% of TS patients, with ADHD and OCD being most common, depression is also common in people with TS, occurring in up to three quarters of patients attending specialist clinics. In published studies, patients with TS are more depressed than healthy subjects (i.e., the person with TS is more vulnerable to depression than a healthy individual). It appears that the depression encountered in people with TS is associated with tic severity and duration, the presence of echo—and copro-phenomena, premonitory sensations, sleep disturbances, OCB/OCD, self-injurious behaviors, aggression, CD in childhood and possibly ADHD (Chapter 3). Depression in people with TS has been shown to result in a lower QOL. The cause appears to be multifactorial (including side effects of medication and a chronic stigmatizing disorder).

SELF-CONCEPT IN AND PUBLIC PERCEPTION (STIGMA) OF PEOPLE WITH TS

Few studies have been published in the area of self-concept in TS, but the results do suggest that some youngsters with TS are no different than healthy "normal" children. However, it may be that severity of TS is associated with TS children's self-reports of behavior disturbance and depressed/irritable mood, although not with overall self-concept. Others suggest that the biggest predictor of psychosocial difficulties in youngsters with TS is the ADHD symptom severity; for children with TS-only, the psychosocial health is no different from the normal general population. Similarly, in adults with TS + high obsessive compulsive symptoms, but not TS-alone ("pure" tics); there is lower self-concept than the general population. Adults with TS and high obsessive compulsive symptoms may have higher social anxiety than the general population, but no differences in public self-consciousness. Once again, people with "pure TS" (i.e., only tics) show no difference from the general population, and only TS+OCB patients had these difficulties. In summary, it appears that it is the *co-morbidity and not the TS per se* that causes difficulties with self-concept in people with TS, be they young people or adults.

It is curious that one may think that people with TS are vulnerable to stigmatization, but public attitudes to TS have seldom been studied. It has been suggested, however, that the single most important factor affecting young people with TS is the *understanding and acceptance* of their family, friends and teachers towards TS. Studies have been undertaken in both schools and universities about the understanding of and stigma towards people with TS. They have shown that knowledge about TS occurred in almost three quarters of school pupils in the USA and half knew that TS was genetic. Over half had a tolerant attitude towards the behavioral difficulties in people with TS, which increased with advancing age and school grades. These attitudes were more positive and comprehensive in families where someone suffered from emotional or psychiatric difficulties. Some folk understood that TS was an emotional and behavioral entity. The majority understood that the disruptive and behavioral outbursts encountered in people with TS are not under the control of the individual. However, others very worryingly felt that the "TS behaviors" should be punished, and as high as a quarter felt that the police should be involved. On a better note, 56.6% were willing to make friends with a person with TS. In a study undertaken in students at a UK medical school, it was shown that more students knew someone with epilepsy than someone with TS. They were more likely to know a public figure with TS. In addition, amongst medical students, a higher proportion has seen someone showing evidence of TS than had seen anyone having a seizure. What is staggering is that as many as a quarter of medical students would *object* to having a son or daughter of theirs marry a person with TS, and around a fifth would object to the marriage of one of their children to a person with epilepsy. It does seem that there is still some stigma towards people with TS and that more public education is needed.

CONCLUSIONS

TS is now recognized to be common, affecting up to 1% of children. In other words, one in a hundred people have TS, although for the vast majority, it is mild and undiagnosed. Just think—you know a hundred people—so you know someone with TS—even if they have not been diagnosed and have mild symptoms. Many individuals with TS (up to 90%) also have co-morbid disorders, NOSI, SIB and thus other problems, which could be described as psychosocial. This may occur in the home with the family, in the community, at school, in areas of entertainment such as the theatre and employment. One of the areas that TS symptoms may not be noticed may be in the sporting arena, as tics generally lessen when the person is playing a sport. It is unclear how many people with TS-only in the community have psychosocial problems, but we just have to look carefully at the stories of professionally successful physicians, such as Dr. Turtle and Dr. Zinner, to see the problems they encountered.

It is therefore clear that TS is more common than it appears, the psychosocial aspects and consequences are frequent, and that many with the disorder may well be disadvantaged and have difficulties. Many of the difficulties of TS are experienced within the individual (e.g., Bliss', Hollenbeck's and Turtle's inner sensations), but many are due to the obvious loud vocal tics and the obvious motor tics, such as the *"possibly offensive"* copropraxia. Others are due to the co-morbidity which occurs in up to 90% of people with TS. Apart from managing and treating the individual with TS, the *education* of the general public, teachers, doctors and employers is of vital importance to improve the psycho-social aspects of the person with TS.

Table 1: Some of the Psychosocial Consequences of Tourette Syndrome at a Glance

Types of Reports in the Literature	Psychosocial Consequences of TS
Case report of Marquis de Dampierre	Ostracised by society and forced to live alone in a tower.
Personal accounts	People with TS have been: Teased, mocked, bullied, and criticised by peers & teachers.
Case reports—side effects of medications	School phobia; separation anxiety.
TS youngsters compared to youngsters with diabetes	TS youngsters have poorer peer relationships than classmates & more than those with diabetes. Psychosocial problems due to TS and *not generic* from chronic disorder.
Community studies	School problems are frequent in youngsters with TS .
Clinical cohorts	One third have social problems.
TS versus TS + ADHD in adults	TS+ADHD individuals have more: Forensic (legal) problems, drug & alcohol abuse, and aggressive behaviour.
Clinical studies including adults & young people	Individuals with TS have a reduced quality of life.
Clinical cohorts TS	Parents of youngsters with TS have increased parenting stress.
Review of literature	TS people are significantly more depressed than control groups. Correlates of depression include tic severity and childhood CD.
Controlled studies	People with TS have a poor psychosocial outcome and the clinical correlates are: = Tic severity = ADHD severity = OCD severity

Table 2. Some Past & Present Famous or Successful People with Tics or TS

Person	Dates	Country/Comments
King William 3rd	1650-1702	England
Peter the Great	1672-1725	Russia
Napoleon	1669-1821	France
Dr Samuel Johnson	1709-1784	England
Dmitry Tolstoy		Russia
	Contemporary famous people with TS	
Perfect Pete		Winner Big Brother UK (TV program)
Kurt Cobain		Rock Star
Julius Wechter		Marimba player (Tijuana Brass)
Mahmoud Abdul-Rauf		Professional NBA basketball player
Tim Howard	Won TSA "Personality of the Year" award 2003	USA, Manchester United, Everton goal-keeper (soccer)

Acknowledgement: The author would like to thank Dr. Petra Kahle for her encouragement and suggestions.

References

1. Carter, A.S., O'Donnell, D.A., Schultz, R.T. & Scahill, L. (2000). Social and emotional adjustment in children affected with Gilles de la Tourette's syndrome: associations with ADHD and family functioning. *J Child Psychol Psychiatry* **41,** 215-223.

2. Cooper, C., Robertson, M.M. & Livingston, G. (2003) Psychological morbidity and caregiver burden in parents of children with Gilles de la Tourette Syndrome (TS) compared with parents of children with asthma. *J Am Acad Child Adolesc Psychiatry* **42(11),** 1370-1375.

3. Cutler, D., Murphy, T., Gilmour, J. & Heyman, I. (2009) The Quality of Life in young people with Tourette Syndrome. *Child Care Health Dev* **35(4),** 496- 502.

4. Eapen, V. & Robertson, M.M. (2008) Clinical Correlates of Tourette Syndrome Across Cultures: A Comparative Study between UAE and UK. Primary Care Companion. *J Clin Psychiatry* **10(2),** 103-107.

5. Elstner, K., Selai, C.E., Trimble, M.R. & Robertson, M.M. (2001) Quality of life (QOL) of patients with Gilles de la Tourette's Syndrome. *Acta Psychiatr Scand* **103,** 52-59.

6. Gorman, D.A., Thompson, N., Plessen, K.J., Robertson, M.M., Leckman, J.F. & Peterson, B.S. (2010) A Controlled Study of Psychosocial Outcome and Psychiatric Comorbidity in Older Adolescents with Tourette Syndrome: a controlled study. *Br J Psychiatry* **197,** 36-44.

7. Haddad, A.D.M., Umoh, G., Bhatia, V. & Robertson, M.M. (2009) Adults with Tourette's syndrome with and without Attention Deficit Hyperactivity Disorder. *Acta Psychiatr Scand* **120(4),** 299-307.

8. Muller-Vahl, K., Dodel, I., Muller, N., Munchau, A., Reese, J.P., Balzer-Geldseter, M., Dodel, R. & Oertel, W.H. (2010) Health Related Quality of Life in Patients with Gilles de la Tourette Syndrome. *Mov Disord* **25(3),** 309- 314.

9. Robertson, M.M. & Cavanna, A.E. (2008) Tourette Syndrome: The Facts. 2nd edition. Oxford University Press, Oxford.

10. Robertson, M.M., Eapen, V. & van de Wetering, B.J. (1995) Suicide in Gilles de la Tourette's syndrome: report of two cases. *J Clin Psychiatry* **56,** 378.

CHAPTER 15

LIVING WITH TOURETTE SYNDROME

Samuel H. Zinner, M.D. and Christine Erdie-Lalena, M.D.

INTRODUCTION

Is TS a disability? Many people have strong feelings about disability, yet may also have trouble defining exactly what the word means. Is the child, adolescent or adult with TS "disabled"? This is an important question to consider. Whether by careful evaluation or through the day-to-day process of simply living life, people with TS are affected by a variety of ideas about disability: their own thoughts about disability in general, and about their place in the world, are shaped in part by how their communities and the greater society view disability. To understand disability at any stage of life in the person with TS, let's start by describing the meaning of disability.

Disabilities are features that interfere with a person doing something as easily as most other people can do. Disabilities can have any or all of three important arms. These three possible parts involve: 1) the person's body and brain; 2) the ability to do something the person wants or needs to accomplish; and 3) the ability to participate with other people. The World Health Organization (WHO) was developed by the United Nations to help to consider disability and other health questions all over the world. In 2001, the WHO improved its definition of disability, and that improvement is helping to change ideas about disability in TS. The WHO said that societies are responsible to make their communities accessible to everybody. What this boils down to is that a society that is completely accessible to everyone will, in effect, eliminate an enormous part of disability. In other words, if everyone is able to participate in everything that society offers, then the experience of disability becomes much smaller.

DISABILITY AND TOURETTE SYNDROME

How do these new definitions of disability apply to living with TS? To answer this, it's helpful to consider what we mean by the name "Tourette". There are several words used in combination with "Tourette", but mostly you will hear "Tourette syndrome" or "Tourette disorder". A syndrome usually describes a group of symptoms that occur together without any mention of whether the symptoms cause any problems. A disorder means that the affected person has difficulties with the symptoms. This means that a syndrome may or may not cause a disability, while a disorder implies a disability. For this chapter, we will stick with the name "Tourette syndrome".

While everyone agrees that no two people are alike, not everyone understands that no two people with TS are alike in how TS affects them. Even if the symptoms of two people with TS look identical to a stranger, parent or teacher, the actual experience of TS for each individual is unique. To complicate matters, most people with TS also have one or more related non-tic problems that accompany TS, as described earlier in this book. And perhaps the most unique part of having TS is how the person lives with it. The question of whether she or he lives with a disability may depend on whether the person is included or excluded from any number of things: from travelling place to place or participating in events at public places, sitting in a classroom at school, finding or keeping a job, being bullied, finding comfort and joy in relationships, and in other ways. The impact on the health and social well-being of the individual most closely defines how that person lives with TS, and if and how that person is disabled.

Importantly, the WHO stated that "mental" disability is every bit as important and real as physical disability. Since tics and many problems that go along with tics come from the brain, TS can be thought of as a mental condition and, for people with TS who are limited by tics or associated challenges, as a mental disability. People with TS may also have physical disability related to their diagnosis. People with TS often cannot participate in everything available in their communities. For example, people with loud or embarrassing tics may be asked to leave public places, like movie theaters or stores. Neighbors may complain about tic noises. A student with TS who also has learning problems may be misunderstood by a teacher who thinks the student is lazy. A person with frequent tics who works as a secretary may find that he is no longer able to type if a new tic develops that makes him slam the keyboard with his palms. People with TS may be teased or bullied about their tics or other behaviors. People with TS may find themselves excluded in these or other ways, and this is why the change in the WHO definition of disability is so important to how people can and do live with TS. The revised WHO definition of disability urges us to find ways to solve or work around these problems as a community so that people with TS are not excluded.

AGES AND STAGES: CHALLENGES WITH TS ACROSS A LIFETIME

Tics usually emerge during a child's first decade of life. However, children with chronic tic behaviors may also have non-tic problems like fidgetiness, impulsive behavior, or social difficulties that may also start early in childhood, well before these children have tics, perhaps as early as infancy and some behaviors perhaps even before birth. Other similar problems can first emerge much later in the life of a person with TS, sometimes not even until adult life, such as depression, anxiety or great difficulty in personal relationships. When these non-tic traits are present, they shape life experience, for better and for worse. The experiences can change with time and maturity. For some people with TS, these traits and experiences result in disability.

At life's beginning, infants and toddlers vary in how patiently and happily they learn and interact with other people. Some babies are very easygoing while others have colic or fussiness, where nothing seems to settle their nerves. We don't yet know if babies who later develop TS symptoms have early life differences as compared to babies who don't develop TS, but they may. Researchers are hard at work trying to find answers to questions like this. We now know that some people cope well with tics and other problems throughout life, even if these people live in very difficult or terrible life conditions. These people are called "resilient". Other people do well only when they are given life conditions that are perfect for their particular needs. Such people are called "vulnerable". People are probably born either resilient or vulnerable, and there seem to be early-life behavior clues that may one day help doctors and others see these differences in people as infants to help prevent later problems for vulnerable children before ongoing struggles begin.

Beyond the toddler years, children with TS are often anxious or nervous. These children may also do things without thinking carefully first. Or, they may have difficulty using their smarts as well as they would like to do. They may struggle to organize their homework or their time, or find that they don't easily blend in with many other kids on the playground or after school.

As these young children grow into teens, their problems can grow with them. New problems may also develop. For example, these teens can develop obsessive thoughts that worry or annoy them, and much as they try, have great difficulty getting these thoughts out of their heads. Teens with or without TS normally sleep differently than young children do, but children and teens with TS may have important kinds of sleep problems that most other young people don't have, like trouble falling or staying asleep. Their tics may also become much stronger or more frequent or, even if their tics don't change much, teens may start to feel very embarrassed about tics that didn't bother them so much when they were younger. Teens may feel excluded because of TS. Some may start smoking or using drugs as a way to fit in, manage stress or avoid unpleasant parts of their life.

As these teens grow into adults, other changes also may occur. Adults with TS seem to be at a higher risk than other adults to become depressed and worried. They may have difficulties in building romantic relationships or in working or even just being comfortable with others. They may also find that some new parts of their world exclude them, such as possible job employers, or even insurance companies that won't provide insurance to adults diagnosed with TS, thinking that TS is somehow too risky a disorder to cover.

LIVING (AND LIVING IT UP) WITH TS: THERE IS A LOT YOU CAN DO!

Whether tic symptoms are mild or severe, whether the tics go away entirely as a child grows or instead last throughout adulthood, whether a person with TS has no other mental or physical challenges or instead has mountains of associated challenges, it is important to strive to live one's life free of having TS symptoms in charge. While this freedom may not mean that symptoms are cured, it does mean that people with TS and those in their lives must find ways to reduce disability associated with their symptoms. A sense of purpose and belonging helps people to thrive. Family and friends help people to do well in life and to feel supported and connected. The ideas and resources below can help direct individuals, families, healthcare providers, educators, policy makers and others on the right path.

IDEAS FOR EVERYONE, NO MATTER WHAT AGE

To start, some ideas can be useful to people of all ages with TS and related conditions.

Tourette Syndrome Association

Take advantage of the information this organization offers to individuals, families, educators and others. Find ideas that allow for inclusion in all aspects of life (tsa-usa.org).

Disabled vs. Differently-abled

Strive to build an identity of ability, rather than of disability. Identify strengths and build on these, using accommodations where needed. Build hobbies that are interesting and challenging. Be creative and hard-working with school or work, be willing to ask for help, and help others where you can.

Medical Home

Find a primary care provider who will partner with you and your family to provide complete care coordination. Specifically, seek out a primary care provider who is interested in developmental, behavioral and social pieces of health and well-being. Recognize that many professionals are not experts in TS. This is OK, provided the professional realizes this, is interested and willing to help, and can assist in finding experts to help provide relevant expertise (medicalhomeinfo.org).

Wraparound

Recognize the lifespan nature of developmental and behavioral differences, and become familiar with "wraparound", which is an intensive process of care to help people with complex needs and their families plan and manage their lives effectively. Wraparound can and should be included in Medical Home partnerships. Wraparound works to solve problems and build skills in coping that are creative and individualized to the child or adult and family (nwi.pdx.edu).

Care Notebook
Develop and maintain a care notebook that can be shared with healthcare providers, educators, and yourself. This type of notebook usually contains pertinent medical documents including primary care providers' notes, laboratory and imaging study results, as well as non-medical documents, such as school reports, etc. (medicalhomeinfo. org/for_families/care_notebook).

If It's Not Broken, Don't Fix It
Tics are not the defining life experience or challenge for many people with TS, and tics usually become less problematic as people with TS grow older. Rather, associated problems and individual strengths and challenges usually determine how one lives with TS.

Self-Esteem
No one single identifiable thing determines self-esteem. Self-esteem can both improve and deteriorate across life stages and circumstances. Pay attention to self-esteem throughout life. Nurture activities, lifestyles and points of view that nurture good self-esteem. A helpful video that broadly discusses nurturing self-esteem from the perspective of one adult with TS is available online at tsa-usa.org/anewmedia/VideoPlayer. html.

Prepare For Life
Life's outcomes and hurdles are surprising and unexpected, mostly filled with unknowns. Whatever the outcomes, work to build safeguards and resiliency rather than preparing for a specific but unpredictable TS or other health-related outcome. Anticipate and become aware of possible future scenarios associated with TS, including maturation patterns. Discover common changes that occur among children with attention deficit hyperactivity disorder (ADHD), for example, as these children mature toward adolescence and then adulthood. Plan to build

skills today that will be as useful now as in the future. For example, people diagnosed with ADHD usually have difficulties in their ability to organize their lives. Young children can learn organizational skills, especially if their families structure the family life in organized ways. As the child grows, the organizational skills can become more sophisticated to reflect the increasingly mature and complicated demands of life. Recognize that some challenges may not be apparent until later in life, such as learning disabilities in abstract language or complex mathematics. Knowing about such challenges before they occur can help you prepare appropriately if and when they do.

Use Symptoms To Your Advantage

Some people with obsessive-compulsive tendencies use perfectionism to excel in their work, studies, and hobbies. These tendencies can be positive attributes. Others with ADHD harness their boundless energy in sports and other interests. There are artists, writers, physicians and others with TS who have identified this trait as key to their success. A well-known painter whose learning disability makes it difficult for him to understand large visual images instead brings together the thousands of tiny pieces that make up a large image, allowing him to paint a remarkably lifelike big picture. A professional musician finds his tic symptoms are absorbed into his piano playing, bringing strength, emotion and character to his music. Several people of all ages have used their experiences with TS to educate others about the disorder, and some have even built their careers around TS education.

Learn Negotiation Skills

Such skills are useful in advocating for oneself. These skills will help in school, in relationships, friendships, at work, for special education accommodations, and in other settings.

Research

Find out about what's happening in TS research. Consider participating in research. The Tourette Syndrome Association and the National Institutes of Health are excellent sources to find out about research activities and opportunities (clinicaltrials.gov).

Sleep

Up to half of all people with TS have disturbed sleep. These difficulties may be caused by other symptoms, like anxiety, or may be caused by differences in how the brains of people with TS organize their sleep. The possible impacts of poor sleeping on thinking, learning and well-being require careful consideration. A useful first-step is to consider good "sleep hygiene". Reference information through the National Sleep Foundation may provide useful insights. Ongoing difficulties should be discussed with one's primary care provider (sleepfoundation.org).

Humor

Laughter is indeed good medicine and humor is useful in bridging relationships with people. Ridicule, humiliation and other bullying behaviors are almost certainly not helpful in building adaptive life skills. However, in appropriate circumstances it is helpful to look at oneself with humor. If done respectfully, and at the right time and place, finding humor even in one's own behaviors that look peculiar or funny to others can be OK, provided the differences between friendly teasing vs. abusive bullying are obvious and agreeable to everyone involved.

IDEAS FOR FAMILIES

Family Dynamics Guidance

TS can be very challenging for affected individuals and for other family members. Difficulties with tic behaviors, impulsive behavior, mood, anger and anxiety can put tremendous strain on families and relationships. The possible impacts of these strains on siblings, between parents and in parent-child interactions should be recognized and monitored. Individuals have different experiences, challenges, perspectives, beliefs and even values within families. Seek help. Online sources of information on a variety of topics in "family dynamics", including communication, discipline, types of family and other topics, are available through the American Academy of Pediatrics at healthychildren.org/English/family-life/family-dynamics/Pages/default.aspx. Professional help with a family-based counselor to improve communication and build positive strategies may improve the family's ability to cope and improve quality of life.

Families As Advocates

Parents can learn methods in assertiveness without using confrontation. Confrontation when arguing for special education services or other purposes may feel fair and it may even feel good. Confrontation may even win "battles", but it probably won't build ongoing trust between families and schools or others, and learning "win-win" strategies in assertive but respectful advocating is a solid investment of a parent's time. Resources to help build effective skills in advocating are available through the Tourette Syndrome Association, Inc. (TSA) at http://www. tsa-usa.org, select the Learn tab, then Education, then Education Advocacy.

Sibling Support

Siblings of people with special needs have unique experiences, challenges, responsibilities and concerns because of their special role in the family. Workshops to help educate families and support siblings can allow opportunities to build skills in advocacy, provide peer support and other benefits siblingsupport.org.

IDEAS DIRECTED TO INFANTS AND TODDLERS

Early Intervention and Prevention

Early Intervention Services are available in all 50 States, providing a variety of services to children from birth to 3 years of age and their families who have or are at increased risk to have a disability. The disability can be physical, "mental" or social and emotional. If found eligible for services, the child and family may receive support for family/parenting training, child development therapies and other supports free of cost. Primary care providers should monitor the child's development, behavior and social environment through routine surveillance and periodic screening and refer for further evaluation if indicated. Children of families with members who have been diagnosed with developmental and behavioral challenges like TS are at increased risk for having developmental and behavioral challenges, too. The National Early Childhood Technical Assistance Center has information and referral support if help is desired nectac.org.

Positive Parenting

No one is born a parent. Becoming a parent under any circumstance is a new and usually stressful experience. There is a lot to learn. Successes and mistakes are part of the plan. All parents should have access to good-quality parenting information from respected sources. Books, classes, videos and websites are popular and useful sources. There are many parenting styles, but most experts agree that Positive Parenting works best in the long run to help children build strong social skills and independence. Positive parents are highly demanding and highly responsive. This style is called "authoritative parenting" (not to be confused with authoritarian parenting). Most popular parenting resources will promote the authoritative parenting style. The American Academy of Pediatrics provides a useful first-stop for parenting information at healthychildren.org/English/Pages/default.aspx

Celebrate Temperamental Differences

In the not-so-distant past, experts thought that children were born with a behavioral "clean slate", and that their behaviors, personality and abilities were molded entirely by the places and people they lived with and around. We now know this belief is not at all true. Some infants are naturally easygoing while others are, by nature, very difficult. Infants don't choose to be easygoing or difficult. Rather, they're born with temperamental and other qualities that determine these behaviors. Research finds there to be nine fundamental temperamental traits. Parents do well to learn about temperamental differences. It's not unusual for a parent and a child to have temperamental styles that are somewhat mismatched to each other. Parents can learn ways to help children with challenging temperaments cope better with stress (including their own).

Smoking

It's not clear whether tobacco exposure to a fetus through a pregnant mother's smoking or chewing tobacco can later affect tics and other related symptoms after birth as the child matures. However, there are many reasons pregnant women should quit smoking. Women who wish to become pregnant or are pregnant can seek help to quit smoking. The American Lung Association offers support lungusa.org/stop-smoking.

IDEAS DIRECTED TO SCHOOL-AGE CHILDREN

Medication Moderation
Several available prescription medications can help reduce tic behaviors, hyperactivity and impulsive behaviors, sleep difficulties, anxiety, obsessions and compulsions, depression and other features. No medication cures TS or non-tic related symptoms. Be careful not to equate "treatment" and "medication". Medications don't teach skills in coping and getting along. However, medication may be part of treatment. Side effects occur with all psychiatric medications. A detailed discussion of medications can be found in Dr. Gilbert's chapter, and further information about non-prescription complementary or alternative interventions can be found in Dr. Kompoliti's chapter.

Tourette Syndrome Overview—Online Video
The Tourette Syndrome Association features an online video presentation in 3 parts, entitled, "Newly Diagnosed". In this video, Dr. Walkup presents a very detailed overview of Tourette syndrome and related problems, including diagnosis and management. The video is an excellent source of information for parents of children with TS, as well as for teachers and healthcare professionals tsa-usa.org/ZNewDiag01/content.html.

Anger Outbursts—Online Video
Anger outbursts may be associated with TS and with associated conditions, including attention deficit disorders, social challenges, and anxiety, among others. Children with Tourette syndrome are at increased risk for associated conditions, and when excessive anger outbursts are part of the picture, further professional evaluation may be indicated to determine whether associated conditions are suspected. In addition to exploring those possibilities, a careful evaluation will consider factors beyond the child that may be contributing to these outbursts. Further discussion of anger in Tourette syndrome can be found in Dr. Budman's chapter. The Tourette Syndrome Association features a brief, excellent discussion with Dr. Walkup entitled, "A Psychiatrist Talks to Parents about Anger" tsa-usa.org/Z_TSA_video/intro.html.

The Play Is The Thing

Children need to play, explore and make believe. Children improve their social skills with practice, trial and error through play, and should be provided with lots of different opportunities in safe and supervised places year-round to do so. The foundations for optimal social skills during adulthood are paved in these early years.

Anxiety

Excessive anxiety is common in TS, and can impair quality of life, function and mood. Children with TS and other family members should be screened for the presence of excessive anxiety or anxiety disorders. Children with anxiety disorders require supportive management that is specific to these diagnoses. Such treatments may include cognitive and behavioral therapy and medication.

Coordination Problems

Visuomotor difficulties are probably more common in people with Tourette syndrome than in the general population. Young children with Tourette syndrome who have visuomotor difficulties may seem clumsy, or have difficulty in learning motor skills, like tying shoelaces, using utensils or holding a pencil easily. These coordination difficulties may predict later problems in severity of tics or problems with well-being as an adult. Young children with fine motor or gross motor developmental difficulties should be followed closely by their primary care providers, families and teachers. If unusual challenges in coordination are suspected, an evaluation with an occupational therapist or other developmental specialist is appropriate. Note that children with these types of coordination problems may be discouraged or excluded from participating in sports or in playing musical instruments. However, if activities like playing sports or a musical instrument are appropriately accommodated, a child may otherwise build better self-esteem and hobbies that can serve as lifelong outlets for social success.

Tourette Syndrome—Video For Families And Others

Collectively, the TSA and HBO channel have produced an Emmy Award-winning program directed to children and adults. The video, titled "I Have Tourette's But Tourette's Doesn't Have Me", presents children with TS from their unique experiences, and methods by which they cope and succeed. A DVD copy of the video is available through the Tourette Syndrome Association tsa-usa.org.

Bullying

Children with behavioral and developmental differences are at higher risk than their typically developing peers to be victimized by bullying behaviors. Adults are often unaware that a child is being bullied, in part because children may feel ashamed. An excellent online resource, using cartoon video clips, is available at http://www.stopbullying.gov. The Tourette Syndrome Association also provides information at tsa-usa. org/educ_advoc/bullying.htm.

IDEAS DIRECTED TO ADOLESCENTS

Anxiety And Mood

Mood disorders (e.g., depression) and anxiety disorders (e.g., excessive worrying, phobias, and obsessions and compulsions) are common among adolescents with TS. Impairments in mood and anxiety can have far-reaching impacts on the youth and others close to her or him. Impacts on quality of life, performance in school, sleep, social behavior and general health may result. Also, anxiety and mood can influence severity or perception of tic behaviors. All people with TS deserve regular professional screening with a primary care provider for anxiety and mood disorders at the top of the list for general healthcare management. Optimal management of TS requires focus on mood and anxiety disorders when present.

Peer Support

Adolescents are usually very aware of how they do or do not fit in with peers. Having behavioral or health-related differences can put teenagers at risk of feeling or being isolated from other teens. These teens may find it helpful to contact other teens who have similar challenges. This form of support can build social bonds and reduce negative feelings about oneself. The Tourette Syndrome Association provides such a source of support.

Youth Ambassador Program

There are unlimited ways to build self-esteem, ability in self-advocacy and excellent communication skills. Some teens with TS can feel that living with their tics and associated problems is awkward or embarrassing. They may find other people to be confused, intolerant or amused by their difficulties. The TSA has taken advantage of a program developed by a teen with TS, called the Youth Ambassador Program, to guide adolescents with TS in helping to educate their peers about this disorder in a friendly and engaging way. The program is available on DVD through the TSA. http://www.tsa-usa.org, select the link to Children & Teens.

Preparing For Transitions

Transitions are a part of life for everyone. Our bodies, minds and lives are always changing in expected and unexpected ways. Children, adolescents and young adults with TS can prepare for these changes by becoming aware of opportunities and challenges to support transitions related to life, work, school, health and other arenas. Useful resources designed for these purposes include Youthhood (youthhood.org) and the National Center on Secondary Education and Transition (ncset. org).

IDEAS DIRECTED TO ADULTS

Mostly For Adults

TS is one of many brain-based conditions that nearly always first becomes apparent in early childhood. However, like many such conditions, TS usually has lifelong symptoms, and many of these symptoms change from childhood to adulthood. Still, most research and services directed in TS focuses on children and youth. Increasingly, physicians, health and social services agencies are recognizing the need to understand adulthood outcomes in TS and related conditions. The TSA provides many online articles to better help adults living with TS understand and balance these issues. This range of topics includes aging with TS, laws regarding airline travel, welfare benefits, health insurance, housing, employment and disability legal rights. Other topics that often first become important in adolescence and young adulthood include dating, military participation, strategies to deal with tics in public, planning for or managing college and living on one's own. The TSA website has a section for adults that talk about these issues. The web link also includes a video presentation on Self-Esteem by an adult with TS who discusses his own strategies in building his self-esteem despite a number of the difficulties he confronts related to TS. He discusses finding personal strengths and building hobbies that allow interaction, taking care before he speaks up about something to research it carefully if he's worried that he may become embarrassed by it, and other strategies. The web link is http://www.tsa-usa.org, select the link to Adults.

Profiles of Adults With TS

The New York Times published an online collection of adult experiences with TS. The collection is titled "Patient Voices". Here, each of these seven adults describes her or his personal experiences with TS. Some of the topics discussed include challenges in sexual intimacy and difficulties with trying to be unnoticed in public when tics are active. The online presentation can be found at nytimes.com/interactive/2010/02/11/ health/healthguide/TE_tourettes.html?ref=health.

Resources

Tourette Syndrome Association Resources:

1.   Tourette Syndrome Association tsa-usa.org

Other Resources:

- Bullying stopbullyingnow.hrsa.gov/kids
- Family Care Notebook medicalhomeinfo.org/for_families/ care_notebook
- Family dynamics healthychildren.org/English/family-life/ family-dynamics/Pages/default.aspx
- Medical Home medicalhomeinfo.org
- National Center on Secondary Education and Transition ncset.org
- National Early Childhood Technical Assistance Center nectac.org
- National Sleep Foundation sleepfoundation.org
- Research activities clinicaltrials.gov
- Sibling support siblingsupport.org
- Wraparound process nwi.pdx.edu
- Youthhood youthhood.org

CHAPTER 16

PARENTING A CHILD WITH TOURETTE SYNDROME

Elaine Fantle Shimberg, B.S.

INTRODUCTION

We all dream of having a perfect child. That's why we count our baby's toes and fingers when he or she is first placed in our arms after the cord is cut. All there! We smile happily. No wonder, then, that it comes as such a shock when that child is seven or eight and we learn that those ever-changing irritating little "habits" we tried to ignore or make excuses for were actually symptoms of a neurological disorder called TS. It's shattering, and no less so when it happens again to one or more of our other children.

Three of our five children, now all adults, have/had Tourette syndrome. I say "had" because although many of their tics were extremely severe as children, they seem to have grown out of them. Fortunately, it sometimes happens but, unfortunately, there's no guarantee that it will.

TAKE TIME TO MOURN

When you first get the diagnosis, you feel numb. It's normal. But the diagnosis also affects the rest of your extended family. Your other children may be embarrassed by their sibling's vocal and motor tics. That doesn't mean your unaffected children don't love their sibling with TS, it just means that being "different" (or having a family member that is) is tough when you're a kid. Grandparents and other family members also may grieve, as well as feel a little guilty for the times they said you needed to punish the child for yelping, or jerking, or other noticeable tics.

"I didn't know," wept one grandmother. "I thought he was just trying to get attention. I feel so badly for what I said."

Said another sadly, "I tried to bribe him to stop sniffing. When that didn't work, I got angry. I thought it was a habit that he could quit if he tried hard enough." While most people seem relieved to finally get a diagnosis to explain what is affecting their child, some parents remain in denial.

"It was better when we didn't know what it was," a mother of a ten-year-old told me. She was convinced TS was a mental disorder and was embarrassed to tell anyone. When I told her it was a neurological disorder, caused by a chemical imbalance in the brain, she felt better. I probably was parroting what the physician originally had told her, but she was not registering the information at that time.

Although I am not a physician, I am a medical writer[1] and a parent of three children who struggled with the symptoms of TS. I also have TS. I have written a number of booklets for the Tourette Syndrome Association, Inc., including booklets for parents, siblings, and grandparents. For these reasons, I am often called by neurologists, psychiatrists, and physicians in my community to speak to and support families and children who have recently been diagnosed with TS.

My advice is often to give yourselves time to get used to the diagnosis, to learn and understand the facts, dispel the myths, and to educate others who are in your child's life, such as other family members, teachers, coaches, religious leaders, and the parents of your child's friends. The good news? Tourette syndrome isn't catching. It also isn't life threatening.

COMMUNICATION

We all can learn ways to improve our communication skills, especially in this era of technological communication with Facebook, texting, e-mails, and blogging. There is nothing like face-to-face communication because it enables us to see body language which, according to a study in the mid-1990s by UCLA's Professor Emeritus, Albert Mehrabian, makes up as much as 93 percent of communication. (That includes 7 percent of meaning in the words that are spoken, 38 percent of the way these words are spoken, and 55 percent in facial expression.) You can't see facial expression or even hear inflection with a text, e-mail, etc. Misunderstandings can and often do happen.

Within your own family, hold regular family meetings. (If you're in a blended family, be sure to include those children who don't live with you full time.) Turn off the TV, collect the cell phones, and let the answering machine take phone calls. It's time to communicate face-to-face.

Often, it is the mother who meets with physicians. If you're the mom, be sure you are quoting the doctors and other professionals correctly. If need be, make an appointment for you all to meet with the doctor. Understand the use of the medications, their purpose, and their possible side effects.

Give everyone in the family an opportunity to express their feelings and concerns. Listen to what they are saying and what they may not be saying. Siblings may worry that they did something to cause their sibling to have TS, or they may resent the attention that sibling is receiving. They may worry about getting TS themselves. One spouse may consciously or subconsciously blame the other. "Didn't you say your grandfather had some type of tics?" while the mother may worry that the one glass of wine she had before she knew she was pregnant could have caused the TS. It didn't!

Reinforce the knowledge that TS isn't a "mental" disorder; it is a neurological disorder. Remind your family that the child's head shaking isn't caused by needing a haircut, the hooting sound isn't a muffled cough from a cold, and the sniffing isn't due to allergies. Educate your family first; then educate the ever enlarging circle.

By communicating with your immediate family first, you prepare them all with the answers to help educate their friends, teachers, employers, and yes, even bullies who sadly inhabit most of our children's worlds. Some children with TS and/or their siblings find that information concerning TS makes a successful "science project" presentation and enjoy being an expert by being able to answer questions from their peers and even their teachers.

BEHAVIOR PROBLEMS

One of the hardest calls to make when your child with TS is acting up is, is this an expression of TS or is it my kid being naughty? The reason it's so difficult is due to the waxing and waning patterns of the tics. It could be a new tic or it could be frustration or depression. It could be an expression of your child's Obsessive Compulsive Disorder (OCD) or Attention Deficit Hyperactivity Disorder (ADHD). It's hard to tell.

A mother told me that her son had stuck his tongue out at his teacher. He was sent to the principal. His parents disciplined him for being rude and disrespectful. Later, however, they saw him sticking his tongue out when he was playing with friends. Yes, it was a new tic, a tongue thrust.

If they had asked him if it was a new tic, he might not have noticed. "I just do it," he said.

Another parent told me that his daughter with TS walked through the family room and knocked over the almost completed 500 piece jigsaw puzzle her siblings had labored over. When asked why she had done it, she replied. "I just wanted to."

"Was it a tic?" he asked. "Did you feel you had to knock it over?"

She thought for a minute. "No, it wasn't a tic. It was me. I think I was mad at them for not letting me help."

It's been my experience that by asking "Was it a tic?" your child knows you trust her to be honest. My kids have lied at times like all kids, but seldom if ever when I asked "Was it a tic?"

Remember the difference between discipline and punishment. Discipline is creating guidelines and rules for behavior; punishment is what happens if the rules are not followed. If you don't create these guidelines and rules for your child because he has TS, you'll have a bratty child with TS. Also rewarding children for positive behavior is a good thing; it is not a bribe. A bribe is rewarding someone for doing something they are not supposed to do.

Kids are smart. They'll play one parent against the other, even more so if parents are divorced. If one or both of you accept any type of bad behavior because "My poor kid has TS and can't help what he does," you'll find that he'll figure anything goes and begin to take advantage of his disorder.

Spend time with your other kids so they don't feel left out. Any chronic disorder like TS affects an entire family and often we are so busy dealing with the problems and needs of our child or children with TS, that we forget these "shadow children" (the other siblings) need our hugs and time alone with us too. I found that riding in the car together with the radio off provided good talking (and listening) time as well as company while getting errands done. Your kids without TS may feel that they caused the TS, because they were mad at their sister or brother and wished something bad would happen. This one-on-one time gives them the opportunity to express how embarrassed they feel from their sibling's tics, anger at the need to defend them from bullies' taunts, and the fear that they too might develop TS. (Never promise that they won't have TS. It has a genetic component, so they might.) One child with TS may complain to you privately about sitting next to a sibling with TS in the movies "because his sniffing makes me want to tic too."

Assure your other children that you understand their frustrations, that sometimes you feel that way too. Encourage them to find ways to cope, such as exercise, music, playing with a pet, etc. Remind them, as my grandmother told me, "Everyone has something and this is what you have." Help them to see past their sibling's TS and learn to accept each other as individuals. Teach them to focus on what's positive and special about each of us.

"HOME" AND "SAFE" ARE GOOD FOUR LETTER WORDS

The tics are part of that child, just as glasses or wheezing from asthma may be with another. When you know what the tics are and accept and work with your child to manage them, the better it will be. You'll quickly learn that your child's tics are more frequent and severe at home than at school or in other public areas. In earlier chapters it was discussed how environments can make tics better and worse. It is important to understand what activities in the home reduce tics and what activities can make tics worse. Planning and structuring your home can make a world of difference for a child with Tourette.

No matter how understandingly planful you can be, the motor movements, shrieks, hoots, and barking noises can wear you down.

It's hard to watch television or have a conversation when these uncontrollable vocal tics keep interrupting. Some families solve the

TV problem by having more than one television or using individual earphones similar to those used on some airplanes.

Motor tics can also present problems. One youngster had an arm tic that caused his arm to swing out. After inadvertently hitting his brother once and on another occasion, breaking a mirror and injuring his hand, his parents suggested that he try to substitute the tic for a hand wave or holding his hands together.

The substitution worked and his parents could once again put pictures on the coffee table and take him out shopping without worrying that he'd break something or knock over a display.

Regardless if you have one child with TS or others with or without it, parents still need some time away from their kids so they can enjoy each other's company as husband and wife and not always Mom and Dad. Obviously, you need to have a qualified and supportive sitter who understands and has been educated about the needs of a youngster with TS. But never underestimate the importance of "getting away." When our five were growing up, we had a standing Wednesday night date. It usually entailed nothing more than a quiet dinner together. The rule (which we broke the first five minutes) was "no talking about the kids."

FACING THE PUBLIC

While the person with TS is surrounded by love at home, going out in public is different. The average person doesn't know or understand what TS is and may think your child is just being naughty and, as I was once told, "You just need to give him a good swat on his behind."

Before going to the grocery or any other public place, ask your child if he or she feels comfortable if you explain TS to others. If so, when your youngster shouts or yelps while you're in the grocery line, just quietly say "I'm sorry if he disturbs you. He has Tourette syndrome and can't control the sounds."

Also, you can have "business" cards printed up for him that say, "I'm sorry if my tics bother you. I have Tourette syndrome."

If the family is going to a movie or the theatre, go at times when there are fewer patrons, or sit in the back so that your child can leave to go to the restroom or lobby for relief if he has to express the tics. Pick restaurants with a private room, or go slightly earlier so that there's less stress on the youngster with TS.

NEVER tell anyone with TS that they can go to the ballet, movies, etc. as long as they don't tic. The stress that scenario creates just makes it almost certain that there will be tics and they'll be stronger and more frequent.

Fatigue also tends to increase the intensity of tics so if you plan a family outing, be sure the child with TS has rested. The day after finals or before starting a new school may not be a good time either. If your youngster doesn't feel like being out in public at a particular time, don't force it. Chances are, he knows how much stress he's feeling and senses it wouldn't be a good time to be with strangers or crowds.

Fortunately, recently there has been a great deal in print and on television about TS so many people have heard of it and will nod and understand. Unfortunately, many of the TV shows still show the person with TS swearing and call it "The Cursing Disease," despite the fact that only about 10 percent of those with TS have that particular tic.

About four years ago, I was contacted by a national talk show. They wanted to have me and my three now adult children on their show. I was pleased to help educate others about TS until the producer said, "What are their tics?"

"Actually," I said, "they have very few at this point, none that you'd notice, in fact. They, like many others, seem to have outgrown the tics."

"None at all?" said the producer. I could hear disappointment in his voice.

"None that you'd notice," I repeated. "It gives hope to many children and their parents who . . ."

But he didn't let me finish. "Television's a visual medium. We need to show what it's like!" And he hung up. Obviously, he needed more education on the subject.

EDUCATION

School can become challenging for a child with TS. The vocal and motor tics create the undesirable in a kid's world; they make him different. It's up to us, the parents, to soothe the path as much as possible by first educating the teachers, librarian, cafeteria workers, the administration, bus drivers, scout leaders, and the coaches. It's time consuming and a never ending job because the personnel often changes from year to year. But without understanding what causes the vocalizations, wiggles, arm

215

thrusts, lack of attention, or kicking, teachers, coaches, and all of the above adults in charge may consider your youngster to be disruptive or trying to be the class clown. A teacher who is educated about TS can not only improve his/her teaching techniques for the child, but also help to prevent or at least, minimize, embarrassment and teasing from classmates.

Unless parents are teachers themselves, it's difficult to understand the myriad acronyms abounding in the academic world. There's the all-important individualized education plan (IEP); learning disabled (LD), important because many children with TS also have OCD, attention disorder disease (ADD), and/or ADHD.

Fortunately, most teachers want all of their students to be successful both academically and socially. That's why they're teachers. (It certainly isn't the "big bucks.")

Make an appointment for both parents, even if you are divorced, to see your child's teacher (s) before school starts or as soon as your child is diagnosed. (An educator confessed to me, "Schools respect seeing both parents.") Bring along some of the excellent material written especially for (and by) teachers, school nurses, and others in the administration from the Tourette Syndrome Association.

If it's a new school, write down what worked before, such as "David was allowed to go to the nurse's office when he felt his vocal tics were getting out of hand," "Sammy does better when he's not sitting in the front row because he knows everyone can see his tics and it makes him self-conscious, stressed, and tic more," or "As Janet's medication makes her tired after lunch, her previous school gave her exams and other stressful work before she ate."

Children with TS usually can keep their tics in check for a short period of time, but when they feel them building, it helps to have a secret code for the teacher to know when the youngsters need to be excused to go out in the hall to express them.

If your child agrees, ask the teacher to talk to the class (when your child isn't there) to explain what TS is and to assure the others that it is not catching. Don't be surprised if the teacher asks you to be there too. Older children may want to talk to their classmates themselves, but never force them to.

It's doubtful that your child is the only student in the class with special needs. The more the classmates learn about TS, about another's child's hemophilia, or another's diabetes, the more they'll learn to be understanding of others and focus on each other's strong points. A caring teacher can educate his/her class about much more than spelling, history, and math.

What if you find the teacher seems resentful of you and your suggestions? Don't get emotional, even though it's difficult when it's your child. One of my daughters, a teacher, admitted, "Teachers talk in the lunchroom, especially about demanding parents."

So think about things from the teacher's viewpoint too. Your child is one of thirty or more kids in the classroom. Many of the students have learning problems, difficulties at home, physical or emotional problems. No wonder most teachers feel over-whelmed. To make it easier, ask how you can help. Volunteer in the classroom? Correct papers? Tutor? Once the teacher knows you're conscious of his or her problems and that you're listening, you may find more cooperation.

KNOW YOUR CHILD'S RIGHTS

In 1975, the United State Congress passed the Individuals with Disabilities Education Act (IDEA). Also known as Public Law 94-142, the Education for All Handicapped Children Act (EAHCA), it says that all children with disabilities have the right to receive "a free, appropriate education." Tourette syndrome IS a handicapping condition under federal law, so your child qualifies in all fifty states. Partial funding for necessary programs comes through the federal government to each state, but in most states, additional funding is local. Unfortunately, that means that special education services vary greatly from state to state and from district to district.

Public Law 94-142 gives parents the right to work with the school in creating a program most beneficial to their child's needs. It also guarantees that your consent must be received before the school can place your child in any program.

All this sounds confusing, but it really isn't. Contact the school's psychologist or administration and let them know that your child has TS and you want an evaluation. There will be a number of diagnostic tests both written and verbal in order to determine various learning problems. It doesn't mean that your child isn't smart. Actually, many children with TS are extremely intelligent and creative. It just means that they learn differently in some cases. It's like having a computer that doesn't "read" specific software so the software has to be customized.

The customized changes for your child are called "accommodations." There are many different ones, including allowing your child to take tests and exams orally rather than written, use a computer, do fewer problems for homework, take tests (even standardized tests) without a time limit, etc.

Children with TS and ADHD often have a long list of cant's in the classroom. They can't sit without fidgeting, can't follow through on instructions, can't finish anything, can't wait their turn, and can't play quietly. As Susan Conners (a teacher with TS and OCD) put it, "To tell parents of these kids that they'd do better in class if they didn't have all of these cant's is like telling the parents of a blind child, 'If your child could see, he'd be a dynamite reader.' It's up to us—teachers and parents—to help that youngster learn coping skills in order to find success in school."[2] Don't be intimidated by all of the academic credentials the psychologists, teachers, and administration have. You have the most important one; you are the parent and you know your child best, so be honest about what you've observed. These professionals are there to help your youngster do well in school.

BULLYING: IT'S TIME TO TALK ABOUT IT

Bullying is the beast in the room that no one wants to talk about. But it's there and as we are now aware, it has invaded cyberspace as well. Many of us experienced bullying as children and were probably told by our parents that the bullies would back down if we stood up to them; easier said than done.

Bullies like targets that are "different" because these differences make those children stand out and make it easy for bullies to make fun of them. It gives bullies a sense of power and control. Certainly, our children's tics set them apart, especially when their peers don't know what causes the movements and vocalizations. That's why it's so important to educate classmates, to let them know that TS isn't catching, the tics are involuntary, and there's no reason to be scared.

Very likely, your kids won't tell you that they're being bullied. They feel ashamed, and embarrassed. Some may even feel that in some way they deserve this treatment. But they don't. No one does. Nevertheless, according to Julie Hertzog, Bullying Prevention Project Director at

PACER (Parent Training and Information Center) and Sandra Hollis, Chair, TSA Education Committee, "reports indicate that over 160,000 children stay home from school every day due to bullying issues."

If your child does tell you about the bullying or you hear it from his or her siblings or a neighbor, what can you do? Encourage your child to:

- Disregard the bully, but don't get angry, scared, or emotional. That's the reaction bullies want.
- Ask the bully to stop: "We don't bully at our school."
- Educate the bully "I have Tourette syndrome. I can't help these tics."
- Move away
- Use humor (if comfortable with it)
- Stay with a peer
- Seek help from an adult; telling isn't tattling

Help your child by doing some role playing, letting them practice different responses; that way a child takes back power and feels more in charge.

Encourage all your children to look out for bullies and to advocate against bullying. According to PACER sources, "Bystanders can make a difference as 60 percent of bullies stop when bystanders interfere." Let bullies know that they aren't wanted in your school, your neighborhood, or on your sports team.

CONCLUSION

Always remember that your child has TS, not you. You need to help by guiding, not guarding. Give them the self-confidence that they are strong and special, that they will be okay in this world.

You'll find that if your child has TS, there will be a lot of both hugs and heartbreak. You don't want them to experience failure, embarrassment, or lack of acceptance. But all of those occurrences are part of life and are learning experiences on which to build coping mechanisms that will carry them into and throughout adulthood. If we somehow prevent our child with TS from any of life's hurts or failures, we keep him or her from learning from them, and even worse, it suggests to our child that we don't think he or she is capable, or is too fragile to cope. Eventually, that youngster will give up trying, figuring that "Mom and Dad don't think I can handle this."

Sadly, we will not always be there to protect our children throughout their lives. And actually, most parents realize this regardless if there's TS or other problems when they have children. It's because we love our kids and whenever they hurt, we hurt too.

I don't know which was sadder for me, to hear of tears and teasing when it actually happened or to learn about it many years later when my adult child finally felt comfortable in telling me.

When I wrote the *Living with Tourette Syndrome* book, I interviewed many children, teenagers, and adults with TS. One of them was a surgeon from Canada who also had OCD.

"How can you operate?" I asked, noticing the way he jerked his arm and then had to 'even it up' by jerking the other.

"I don't tic when I operate," he said simply.

Trying to phrase my question without offending, I stammered, "But how do you get them to lie down on the table?"

The doctor smiled. "They trust me."

And that's the key to raising kids with TS. Let them know in words and deeds that you trust them, you trust them to succeed in their own way.

Acknowledgement: Elaine Fantle Shimberg is an award winning author of twenty-two books, most of which are on health and family issues. She has served on the national TSA board and is past chairman of St. Joseph's Hospital in Tampa, Florida. She is a member of the American Society of Journalists and Authors and the American Medical Writers Association. In 2002, Shimberg was awarded an Honorary Doctor of Humane Letters degree from the University of South Florida. She is the mother of five adult children and has ten grandchildren.

References

1. Shimberg, E.F. (1995) *Living with Tourette Syndrome.* Simon & Schuster, NY.

2. Shimberg, E.F. (1995) *Living with Tourette Syndrome.* p. 161. Simon & Schuster, NY.

CHAPTER 17

HISTORY AND RESEARCH INTO TOURETTE SYNDROME

Kevin St. P. McNaught, Ph.D.

INTRODUCTION

In 19th century France, discoveries in the field of neurology were frequent and impressive. This was, to a great extent, attributed to the brilliance of Jean-Martin Charcot (1825-1893) who is often considered to be the father of modern neurology[1]. While working at the famous Salpêtrière hospital in Paris, France, Dr. Charcot studied and lectured on nervous system disorders, and attended to patients with a wide range of neurological illnesses[1]. He later became director of the Salpêtrière hospital and his strong reputation in neurology attracted many students, including Georges Albert Édouard Brutus Gilles de la Tourette, whom he would train and mentor (Fig. 1).

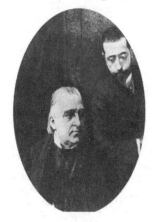

Figure 1. Photograph of (right) Georges Albert Édouard Brutus Gilles de la Tourette (1857-1904) and (left) his mentor, Jean-Martin Charcot (1825-1893).

GILLES DE LA TOURETTE AND MALADIE DES TICS

Gilles de la Tourette was born on October 30, 1857, in the small town of Saint-Gervais-les-Trois-Clochers, France[2]. Little is known about his early life, but he began his medical studies during 1873-1876 in Poitiers and Paris, France. In 1884, Gilles de la Tourette began training under Dr. Charcot's guidance at the Salpêtrière hospital.

Initially, Gilles de la Tourette studied various medical conditions, such as hysteria, hypnosis and ataxia, all of which were of interest to his mentor. Later, however, Dr. Charcot asked him to turn his attention to paroxysmal movement disorders which are neurological illnesses characterized by sudden outbursts of emotion and/or action. It was at this point in his career in 1884, while still being in training, that Gilles de la Tourette probably first encountered the disorder that now bears his name.

In his most famous article, published in the January 1885 issue of the medical journal *Archives de Neurologie*[3], and at the age of 28 years old, Gilles de la Tourette described a bizarre neurological condition that he referred to as "maladie des tics." The article was based on the observation of 9 individuals with a condition that had various features, including childhood-onset, hereditability, waxing and waning, stereotyped movements, premonitory sensation, echolalia and coprolalia. Gilles de la Tourette speculated that the disorder had a degenerative cause wherein the afflicted inherited a nervous system that was weakened by the immoral behaviors of previous generations. Dr. Charcot later renamed the disorder in honor of his student, Gilles de la Tourette, and is now widely referred to as Tourette syndrome (TS) or Tourette disorder (TD).

DEMISE OF A BRILLIANT NEUROLOGIST

It is thought that Gilles de la Tourette qualified as a doctor around 1886, soon after his famous publication on the disorder now named after him. He continued to work on hypnotism, hysteria, neurological conditions and experimental therapies at a number of institutions where he held various positions[4]. He also wrote extensively and published a wide range of medical and other matters of personal interest (e.g. art, literature and law)[4].

Gilles de la Tourette was a highly driven, multi-talented and brilliant scholar of medicine. However, he was often considered to be unstable, irascible, hyperactive and combative. Indeed, he was described by a friend, Paul Legendre, as follows: "So he was a jovial, exuberant chap with an arrogant, unsubtle way of speaking; the voice, unfortunately, was rough and a little hoarse. Very fervent, but with little patience, he was not the man to allow his opponents to let their arguments be taken up and refuted point by point; he got worked up at the first contradiction; even the number of his adversaries did nothing to moderate his reactions and one could hear, in the middle of noisy discussions, the raucous explosions of his overworked larynx."[2].

Tragically, in 1893, both Gilles de la Tourette's son and his mentor, Jean-Martin Charcot, died. During that very same year, Gilles de la Tourette was shot in the head, but not killed, by an apparently psychotic woman (Rose Kamper) who claimed that she had been hypnotized at the Salpêtrière hospital and was now incapable of making a living. Ironically, Gilles de la Tourette himself later developed psychiatric (probably depression and dementia) and neurological (neurosyphilis) illnesses and, in 1901-1902, he was forced to leave his hospital appointment and was admitted to a hospital for mental illnesses in Lausanne, Switzerland. His condition deteriorated significantly and shortly thereafter he died on May 22, 1904.

WAS TOURETTE SYNDROME DESCRIBED PREVIOUSLY?

It is noteworthy that, while Gilles de la Tourette is credited with the discovery of the disorder that bears his name, there is evidence to suggest that this condition was previously described by other clinicians[1,5]. Notably, Jakob Sprenger and Heinrich Kraemer in their book, published in 1498 and entitled "Maleus maleficarum (Witches hammer), described a priest who had motor and vocal tics that were thought to be the result of possession by the devil, witchcraft, or exorcism[6]. In 1825, a French doctor, Jean Marc Gaspard Itard (1775-1838), reported that the Marquise de Dampierre, an important woman of the Parisian aristocracy, suffered from a disorder that was characterized by involuntary movements associated with sudden vocalizations and outbursts of obscenities[7]. Incidentally, she was one of the 9 patients that Gilles de la Tourette described in his 1885 publication on the disorder. An 1873 publication of the famous French physician Armand Trousseau's (1801-1867) monograph also described several patients with motor and vocal tics[8].

Interestingly, Gilles de la Tourette in his 1885 publication briefly mentioned and was mildly critical of Trousseau's earlier observations. Moreover, Hughlings-Jackson (1835-1911), an English neurologist, reported in Clinical Lectures and Reports to the London Hospital a single case of the disorder in 1884[9]. Despite these earlier reports of tics, it was Gilles de la Tourette who clearly reported the many features of the condition and thus he set the stage for the recognition of TS as a distinct neurological disorder. Indeed, given that Gilles de la Tourette was a junior and relatively inexperienced at that time, it is likely that the study and description of the cases presented in the 1885 article were to a great extent the work/influence of his mentor, Dr. Charcot.

THE EMERGENCE OF RESEARCH AND MILESTONES IN TS

Following Gilles de la Tourette's death and up to the early 1960s, there was relatively little interest in studying TS compared to other neurological conditions such as Parkinson's disease and Alzheimer's disease, which were recognized as medical conditions during the same period. This began to change in the 1960s-1970s when Shapiro and colleagues demonstrated that the neuroleptic drug haloperidol could be useful in treating TS symptoms[10]. This observation began to call into question the psychosocial/psychoanalytic view (e.g., having tics relates to sexual feelings and expressions) and the approach to treating the disorder which was proposed by the Hungarian psychoanalyst Sandor Ferenczi (1873-1933) in 1921 and which had prevailed during the previous decades[11].

The establishment of the national Tourette Syndrome Association, Inc. (TSA) in the US in 1972 coincided with, and stimulated significant interest in the disorder during the 1970s and subsequent decades. Indeed, the provision of research grant awards by the TSA (beginning in 1984) and later other organizations across the world served to encourage many research scientists and clinicians to investigate the causes and to seek improved treatments for the disorder (Fig 2.). These efforts have led to breakthroughs in many areas of TS (Fig. 3). Notably, there has been much progress in our understanding of the complex symptomology, progression and the prevalence of TS in the US and worldwide. In addition, although we do not yet have a good understanding of its cause, research has uncovered evidence to suggest that gene mutations and alterations in the basal ganglia play a key role in the development of the disorder. Clinical studies have led to the introduction of various drugs for people with TS. More recently, there has been encouraging developments with behavioral and surgical (deep brain stimulation) therapeutic approaches for the disorder.

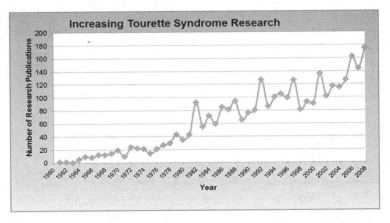

Figure 2. The consistently increasing level of research into TS from the 1960s to 2008. The graph shows the number of publications on Tourette syndrome per year. Data obtained from PubMed.

THE FUTURE OF TS

It is now over 125 years since Gilles de la Tourette clearly described the disorder that now bears his name. Although research into the condition was delayed for many decades, interest began to increase from the 1960s and, today, there are intense investigations into most aspects of the disorder. Significant progress has been made in many of these areas[12]. However, there remain many mysteries and unmet needs in TS[12]. For example, the cause(s) and brain changes underlying the disorder remain unknown. There continues to be a lack of highly effective medications that are devoid of numerous and/or severe adverse effects that often limit the use of current drugs and safe medications for many people with the condition. Therefore, in the years ahead, research will likely focus on these and other unmet needs and unanswered questions in the disorder. Ultimately, we hope that future research will increase our understanding of TS, improve the ability of care providers to manage the disorder, and possibly produce cure for individuals who develop the condition.

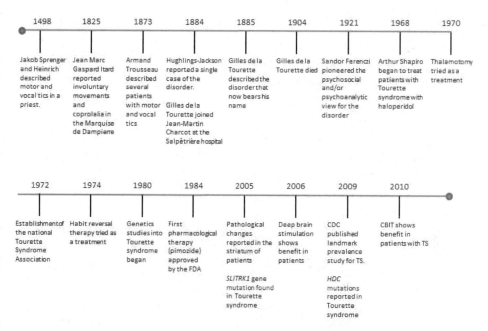

Figure 3. A timeline that shows key discoveries and advances in Tourette syndrome

References

1. Teive, H.A.G., Chien, H.F., Munhoz, R.P. and Barbosa, E.R. (2008). Charcot's contribution to the study of Tourette syndrome. *Arq Neuropsiquiatr* **66**, 918-921.
2. Rickards, H. & Cavanna, A.E. (2009). Gilles de la Tourette: The man behind the syndrome. *J Psychosomatic Res* **67**, 469-474.
3. de la Tourette G.G. (1885). Étude sur une affection nerveuse caractérisée par de l'incoordination motrice accompagnée d'écholalie et de coprolalie. *Arch Neurol* **9**, 19-42, 158-200.
4. Walusinski, O. & Duncan, G. (2010). Living his writings: The example of neurologist G. Gilles de la Tourette. *Mov Disord* **25(14)**, 2290-2295.
5. Goetz, C.G., Chmura, T.A. & Lanska, D.J. (2001). History of Tic Disorders and Gilles de la Tourette syndrome: Part 5 of the MDS-sponsored history of movement disorders exhibit, Barcelona, June 2000. *Mov Disord* **16**, 346-349.
6. Finger, S. (1994). Some movement disorders. In: Finger, S. (ed). Origins of neuroscience: the history of explorations into brain function. New York: Oxford University Press, pp. 220-239.
7. Itard, J.M.G. (1825). "Mémoire sur quelques functions involontaires des appareils de la locomotion, de la préhension et de la voix". *Arch Gen Med* **8**, 385–407.
8. Rickards, H., Woolf, I. & Canvanna, A.E. (2010). "Trousseau's disease:" A description of the Gilles de la Tourette syndrome 12 years before 1885. *Mov Disord* **25(14)**, 2285-2289.
9. Hughlings-Jackson, J. (1884). Clinical lectures and reports to the London hospital. 1452.
10. Shapiro, A.K. & Shapiro, E. (1968). Treatment of Gilles de la Tourette's Syndrome with haloperidol. *Br J Psychiatry* **114**, 345–350.
11. Kushner, H.I. (1999) A cursing brain: the histories of Tourette syndrome. Harvard University Press, MA.
12. McNaught, K. St.P. & Mink, J.W. (2011) Advances in understanding and treatment of Tourette syndrome. *Nat Rev Neurol* **7(12)**, 667-676.

CHAPTER 18

FREQUENTLY ASKED QUESTIONS AND ANSWERS ABOUT TOURETTE SYNDROME

CONTENT

1. What is Tourette syndrome?

Gilles de la Tourette syndrome is a chronic neuropsychiatric disorder characterized by the presence of involuntary motor and phonic tics that wax and wane. In addition to tics, individuals with Tourette syndrome often have a variety of concomitant psychopathologies, including obsessive-compulsive disorder (OCD), attention-deficit hyperactivity disorder (ADHD), learning difficulties, and sleep abnormalities. Although the presence of neurobehavioral problems is not required for the diagnosis of Tourette syndrome, their clinical impact on the patient may be more significant than the tics themselves.

Tics, the essential component of Tourette syndrome, are broadly defined (involuntary, sudden, rapid, repetitive, or non-rhythmic stereotyped movements or vocalizations) and readily observable. They are manifested in a variety of forms with different durations and degrees of complexity, and no two patients have exactly the same symptoms. Simple motor tics are brief, rapid movements that often involve only one muscle group and may include eye blinks, head jerks, or shoulder shrugs. Complex motor tics may be non-purposeful (facial or body contortions) or seem to be purposeful but actually serve no purpose (touching, smelling, jumping, or obscene gestures) or have a dystonic character. Simple vocal tics include sounds such as grunting, barking, yelping, and throat clearing. Complex vocalizations include syllables, phrased, echolalia (repeating other people's words), palilalia (repeating one's own words), or coprolalia (utterance of obscene words). Despite the public's perception of Tourette syndrome, Coprolalia actually occurs in less than 10% of patients.

(Harvey Singer, M.D.; 10 Most Commonly Asked Questions About TS; The Neurologist; Vol. 6, No. 5; September 2000)

2. Is TS a neurological, psychiatric or neurobehavioral disorder?
One of the problems with the term "psychiatric" is that our society is not over the stigma of mental illness. Because of this stigma, some people shy away from the idea that TS is in any way psychiatric. Evidence compiled from neuroimaging and examination of brain tissue of patients with TS after death suggests that the division between neurological and psychiatric may not be as sharp as once believed. In keeping with this view, some suggest the term neuropsychiatric. This term implies that there are both neurological and psychiatric elements in TS.

There is a large body of evidence showing that tics are due to subtle disruption of specific nerve pathways in the brain. Not surprisingly, these nerve pathways have to do with motor action. In order for us to carry out everyday activities or even specialized activities like playing an instrument or hitting a baseball, we have to activate certain muscle groups and deactivate other muscle groups that aren't needed for that action. Thus, coordinated motor action requires facilitation and inhibition of muscle groups at the same time. This coordination is managed by motor pathways in the brain. The involuntary performance of a tic may be a disruption of this balance between facilitation and inhibition of motor pathways. Taken together, this suggests that tics are neurological. But there may be a little more to it.

Careful observation by parents and individuals with TS indicates that tics occur in some situations more than others. Stressful situations, excitement (the Disneyland effect) and anxiety can increase tics. Motor activities involving high levels of concentration (playing the piano) can decrease tics. Recent success with habit reversal training suggests that people can learn techniques to alter or eliminate tics. These observations indicate that environmental factors and learning can influence tics. If environmental factors and learning can influence tics, maybe the term "neurological" is incomplete and that TS may be a bit more complicated than this term implies.

What about the term—neurobehavioral? As many parents of children with TS know, TS is often more than just tics. Children with

TS are more likely than the general population to have problems with impulsiveness, over-activity, distractibility, disruptive and defiant behavior, repetitive behavior and anxiety. Some children with TS have lowered capacity for managing frustration and may over-react to what others consider minor frustration. It is not clear that these problems are part of TS—indeed not every child with TS has such problems. When present, however, these behavioral problems can be far more pressing than tics. Thus, neurobehavioral seems to fit—but consensus on what it means has not emerged.

In conclusion, TS is fundamentally a neurological disorder. Although it is defined by the presence of motor and vocal tics, to say that TS is only neurological suggests that it is only about motor and vocal tics. It is clear that environment influences behavior—including tics. Behavior also influences the environment. Children with TS who are impulsive, disruptive and defiant can pose a real challenge for parents. To promote optimal development for these children with TS, families and clinicians need to look beyond the tics.

(Lawrence Scahill, M.S.N, Ph.D.; Inside TSA; Fall 2009)

3. **Should I be seeing a neurologist or a psychiatrist to treat my TS? I have been hearing different advice from people, and I'm not sure which kind of doctor would be the best for seeking treatment.**

Fortunately, neurologists and psychiatrists, as well as some pediatricians and family practice doctors, can possess the necessary knowledge and skills to care for individuals with TS. So in that sense, a physician's specialty may not be the main fact to consider when choosing a doctor. Therefore, depending on where you live, recommendations may vary as to which doctor might be better qualified. I would suggest that you review the TSA Physician List to identify names of physicians in your area, and then attempt to obtain more information from others as to the strengths and weaknesses of available practitioners. A good source for finding out more may be your local TSA Chapter. Also, many university or regional medical centers have specialty clinics which focus on the needs of patients and families with TS. A bit of extra research can well lead you to a knowledgeable clinician.

(James T. McCracken, M.D.; Inside TSA; Fall 2008)

4. How is the diagnosis of TS made?

Diagnosis is made by observing symptoms and/or evaluating a description of the movements and their onset. Blood tests or other types of neurological testing cannot confirm a diagnosis of TS. However, some medical professionals may order such tests to rule out other conditions that might be confused with TS

(John T. Walkup, M.D.; Questions and Answers about Tourette Syndrome; May 2006)

The diagnostic criteria for Tourette Syndrome as currently established by the Diagnostic and Statistical Manual of Mental Disorders (DSM) 4th Edition, Text Revision requires that both multiple motor and vocal tics be present for a period of time—although not necessarily concurrently, and also that symptoms have to have begun before the age of 18.

Physicians ask about when they can observe the movements and try to learn whether the tics experienced are sudden, rapid, non-rhythmic, recurrent stereotypic movement and/or include vocalizations. Tics typically occur in bouts that are nearly every day or intermittently throughout a period of at least one year or more. A diagnosis requires that the person be without any tic-free intervals for more than three consecutive months. Also, it needs to be assessed whether these symptoms cause distress or significant impairment, and that they cannot be attributed to another underlying physiological problem. Often these tics will be manifested in one area of the body (usually the face or head), will wax and wane in severity and even appear in different parts of the body.

(Cathy L. Budman, M.D.; Inside TSA; Summer 2009)

One really important thing to determine is whether a symptom is actually a tic. One feature that provides a clue that we're dealing with a tic disorder is to ask about premonitory sensations—an itch, an urge, a certain tension felt somewhere in the body that is experienced just before the onset of the tic. The reported presence of these urges can help when firming up the diagnosis. It is sometimes said that these sensations do not occur in young children. However, I have seen some very eloquent children as young as five or six who claim that they feel "an eyelash in my eye and must get it out" before an eye tic. While this phenomenon is not necessary to confirm a diagnosis and some people never report feeling these sensations, nevertheless, describing these premonitory urges can provide support when determining a TS diagnosis.

(Jeremiah M. Scharf, M.D., Ph.D.; Inside TSA; Summer 2009)

5. Please define the differences between a Transient Tic, Provisional Tic, Chronic Motor Tic, or regular Tic Disorder and Tourette Syndrome.

These labels come from the Diagnostic and Statistical Manual of Mental Disorders, Fourth Edition (DSM-IV) published by the American Psychiatric Association. This professional group has tried to set down guidelines for making diagnostic determinations across a wide range of conditions. The term "Tic Disorder" is a general term including: Transient Tic Disorder, Chronic Tic Disorder and Tourette syndrome. The distinction between these labels is related to the type and duration of the tic symptoms.

Transient Tic Disorder is used when motor tics, vocal tics (or both) are present for more than two weeks—but less than one year. Chronic Motor Tic Disorder is the right diagnosis when motor tics—and only motor tics—have been present for at least a year. Although it appears to be less common, Chronic Vocal Tic Disorder is defined by the presence of vocal tics (but no motor tics) for more than a year. The diagnosis of Tourette syndrome requires the presence of multiple motor tics and at least one vocal tic for at least a year.

In addition to the tics for more than a year, the diagnosis of TS requires that the tics be persistent (occurring daily) and there is no significant period of time when the tics are not present. As a guide, the DSM specifies three months, but this period of time is somewhat arbitrary. The intent is to confirm that the person has had an enduring pattern of tics that lasted at least a year.

This can become an issue in the clinic. For example, consider the case of an 8-year-old boy who started having tics at age 6. The parents recall the onset of eye blinking that "lasted for a few months and went away." Sometime later, the child showed facial grimacing—again lasting a few months and then subsiding. At age 7 several other tics appeared. These tics occurred daily and this time they didn't subside. By 8, he comes into the clinic with an enduring pattern of tics lasting six months. His original tics were noticed two years earlier, but were not enduring. Does this child have TS? The answer is probably. But if the diagnostic criteria were strictly applied a little more time would be needed to confirm the diagnosis.

(Lawrence Scahill, Ph.D.; Inside TSA; Fall 2009)

6. **Typically, when do TS symptoms begin? Are there cases that occur in very young children, older teens, and adults? Is it possible to start showing signs of TS later on as well?**

In most cases, the onset of tics occurs between 2 and 15 years of age, with the mean age of onset being seven. Therefore, although more often the symptoms start later, it is not unusual for onset to begin at three. The initial tics usually occur in the upper body, commonly involving the eyes (e.g. blinking) or other parts of the face. Vocal tics usually develop afterward-even one to two years later. Typically, the tics wax and wane with a changing repertoire over time. For the majority of individuals, the period of the worst tics usually occurs between the ages of 7 and 15, and then often there is a steady decline in symptoms. During late adolescence and early adulthood symptoms stabilize, i.e. fewer varieties of tics appear and they are, in many cases, milder. Complete remission of both motor and vocal tics has been reported. However, estimates vary considerably, with some studies reporting rates of remission as high as 50%.

(Katie Kompoliti, M.D.; Inside TSA; Spring 2003)

7. **Everything that I have read says TS symptoms decrease when people reach their 20's. After I turned 30, my tics exacerbated. Is this a common occurrence and will the tics decrease over time?**

In general, tics do lessen gradually after puberty. This observation is not new. Experienced clinicians, parents, and adults with TS have reported this for many years, and two studies conducted at Yale over the past decade have confirmed these claims. These findings suggest that after the onset of tics between the ages of 5 and 7 years, tics follows a fluctuating course with an upward trend until about age 11 or 12. Following this peak severity at age 11 to 12, tics tend to decline. By age 18, most individuals report milder tics than they experienced during peak severity at age 11 or 12. This pattern appears to be true for most, but certainly not all, people with TS.

There are a couple of interesting points to be made about these studies. First, the severity of tics in childhood is only modestly predictive of tic severity in adulthood. For example, children with prominent tics in childhood may still show the typical downward trend already described and go on to show mild tics in adulthood. Only a minority of cases show prominent tics in childhood and continue at that level in adulthood. More rarely, others may have milder tics in childhood and, for reasons that are not clear, have more frequent symptoms in adulthood. Second, is the matter of the overall outcomes of young adults with TS. Tic severity in childhood does not seem to have bearing on overall outcomes such as education, occupational achievement, and family life. However, the presence of ADHD or prominent OCD in childhood appears to be associated with lower educational and occupational achievement regardless of tic severity. This observation suggests that families, school personnel, and clinicians should be especially attentive to ADHD and OCD in children and adolescents with TS.

Because tics do generally decline by early adulthood, we try to think carefully when consulting with patients who report worsening tics in adulthood. In some cases, their history suggests a possible explanation for the worsening of tics. In others, we can't identify a reason for the departure from the usual course of TS. Possible explanations that have been suggested include emerged in exposure to extraordinary life stress and serious cocaine abuse. We have also seen a few cases including body builders who reported increased tics following intensive use of anabolic steroids. I hasten to add that these explanations are educated guesses, and don't explain most TS cases with a worsening of tics in adulthood. Finally, in answer to your question about what to expect from here—it is difficult to predict. Just because your tics have worsened in adulthood, we still do not consider TS to be a progressive disease. Therefore, there is no reason to conclude that your tics will continue to show a steady worsening.

(Lawrence Scahill, Ph.D.; Inside TSA; Summer 2007)

8. **I recently met an adult with TS who was just diagnosed. I was under the impression that TS has to be present during childhood. Are there any exceptions to this? What causes an adult onset of TS or tics? Can this happen due to taking certain medications or could it be related to another medical condition?**

Although Tourette syndrome is considered a childhood-onset disorder, it often persists into adulthood. In a recently published study done to draw attention to and correct the common misconception that TS only occurs in children, the mean age at initial visit of 43 adult TS patients was 59 years. The adult patients were compared to 100 children with TS, who at the time of their visit to Baylor College of Medicine Movement Disorder Clinic, were about 13 years old. Of the adult TS patients, 35 (81.4%) had a history of tics with onset before age 18, with 8 (18.6%) reporting first occurrence of tics after age 18 (mean age at onset 38 years). Only 2 (4.7%) patients reported tic onset after age 50. During the course of TS in the adult patients, phonic and complex motor tics, self-injurious behaviors, and ADHD gradually improved, but facial, neck and trunk tics persisted. Additionally, adults with TS were more likely to exhibit substance abuse and mood disorders compared to children with TS. Although adult TS largely represents re-emergence or exacerbation of childhood-onset TS, there are certain causes of tics that start in adulthood that a neurologist must consider and exclude. These include certain drugs, such as amphetamines and cocaine, and various drugs (also called neuroleptics) used for psychiatric and gastrointestinal disorders (so-called "tardive tics"). Other causes of adult tics include Huntington disease, neuroacanthocytosis (a human brain disease) and a variety of other neurological disorders. Published reports of secondary tics (also called "Tourettism") are referenced in this study (Jankovic J, Gelineau-Kattner RN, Davidson AL Tourette's syndrome in adults. Mov Disord 2010;25:2171-5).

(Joseph Jankovic, M.D.; Inside TSA; Spring 2011)

9. **Besides tics, what other problems may occur in patients with Tourette Syndrome and do these occur with everyone that has TS?**

Comorbid or associated, neuropsychiatric problems are relatively common in individuals with tic disorders. The incidence of obsessive-compulsive behaviors (OCBs) in patients with Tourette syndrome is typically reported to be 40% to 50%, although some studies report an incidence of up to 60% to 89%. Obsessive behaviors generally emerge several years after the onset tics, usually during adolescence. In patients with Tourette syndrome, OCBs usually include a need for order or routine and a requirement for things to be symmetrical or "just right." Hence, compulsions typically involve arranging, ordering, hording, touching, tapping, rubbing, counting, checking for errors, and "evening-up" rituals (performing activities until things are symmetrical or feel and look just right). It has been suggested that simple tics, complex tics, and compulsions represent a clinical spectrum of symptoms in Tourette syndrome, with complex tics and compulsions sharing many overlapping features. There is evidence for a genetic association between OCD and Tourette syndrome; however, OCD is etiologically heterogeneous, and not all cases are associated with a chronic tic disorder.

ADHD is characterized by impulsivity, hyperactivity, and a decreased ability to maintain attention. The disorder is common in Tourette syndrome probands and is reported to affect about 50% of referred Tourette syndrome cases. ADHD typically begins at about 4 to 5 years of age, and in Tourette syndrome patients, it usually precedes the onset of tics by 2 to 3 years. Its appearance is not associated with the concurrent severity of tics, although ADHD is common in patients with more severe tic symptomatology. Whether a genetic relationship exists between Tourette syndrome and ADHD remains controversial. Several studies have found an increased incidence of anxiety and depression in patients with Tourette syndrome. Some investigators believe that depression correlates positively with earlier onset and longer duration of tics, whereas others find no correlations between depression and number of tics. Rage attacks and difficulty with aggression have been described in patients with Tourette syndrome. However, whether these problems as are etiologically related to Tourette syndrome or other comorbid conditions is under review. A variety of other behavioral and emotional problems have been identified in patients with Tourette syndrome. For example, in studies based on the Child Behavior Checklist, up to two thirds of subjects with Tourette syndrome had abnormal scores with clinical problems including OCBs, aggressiveness, hyperactivity, immaturity, withdrawal, and somatic complaints.

(Harvey Singer, M.D.; 10 Most Commonly Asked Questions About TS; The Neurologist; Vol. 6, No. 5; September 2000)

10. Many people with TS develop one or more co-morbidities. What is the time course of the most prevalent of these conditions? In particular, when do OCD, ADHD and/or depression typically first appear, how do they progress over time and do they recede or worsen during adulthood?

Clinically referred youth with TS are often diagnosed with co-morbid psychiatric disorders, which typically emerge during childhood, although their timing and expression can be highly variable. ADHD and OCD are more likely than tics to persist into adulthood, and to be associated with more functional impairment and impact on quality of life. In general, adults with TS are more likely than children to present with obsessions and compulsions, mood disorders and a history of self-injurious behaviors.

Half or more of children with TS evaluated in clinical settings also meet criteria for Attention Deficit Hyperactivity Disorder (ADHD), with symptom onset usually preceding tic onset. ADHD symptoms are usually persistent, although past or current tics appear to have little impact on ADHD outcome. Learning disabilities and executive dysfunctions are generally reported to persist, although long-term outcomes are variable and complicated, with limited available data.

Obsessive-compulsive disorder (OCD) is diagnosed in approximately 20-40% of children who come to a clinic for TS; however, up to 90% may have some obsessive or compulsive symptoms. OC symptoms (OCS) may develop before, simultaneously with, or after onset of tics; OCS frequently emerge or intensify in early adolescence, while the impact of tics usually diminishes. Qualitative adult outcome of those with persistent OCB/OCS may be associated with social anxiety and poor self-esteem.

Much less is known about the onset and course of mood and non-OCD anxiety disorders in TS, although they also frequently co-occur. Generalized anxiety and mood disorders tend to persist, perhaps even in most adults with TD, and may impose a significant toll on functional outcome.

Overall, psychiatric comorbid disorder outcomes are generally thought to be semi-independent of tic outcomes. However, a recent study of older adolescents with TS reported that compared with healthy controls, individuals with TS had significantly higher rates of ADHD, learning disorder, conduct disorder and major depression. In the individuals with TS, poorer psychosocial outcomes were associated with greater ADHD, OCD and tic severity. Although much of the impairment was attributable to ADHD, this study was the first to report that individuals with TS were more likely to develop other psychiatric disorders (except OCD) and major depression, independent of ADHD.

(Barbara J. Coffey, M.D.; Inside TSA; Fall 2011)

11. Some Individuals with TS may develop depression and other co-morbidities that affect their social well-being. Are these co-morbidities a direct result of having to deal with underlying tics or are they independent entities?

Studies have reported a greater lifetime risk for depression in individuals with TS, but data has largely been lacking on the nature and etiology of this association. Some authors have suggested the reason for this association is a possible genetic relationship between tics and depression, and others have conceptualized this association as a function of living with a chronic illness, which can be extremely stressful and debilitating. Others have suggested that there is likely to be a multifaceted interaction between lifetime stress and genetic vulnerabilities.

Some data have suggested that a complex interaction between tic severity, ADHD, OCD and psychosocial stress renders individuals with TS more likely to develop depression. However, the most recent study of older adolescents with TS reported that major depression was the only co-morbid disorder for which there was no association with a lifetime diagnosis of OCD, ADHD or any measure of ADHD, OCD or tic severity. This association remained robust after controlling for the presence of ADHD diagnosis and severity. This finding, which is the first to suggest a possible innate or biological link between TS and depression, raises some interesting new questions, and requires additional research.

People with TS often have anxiety, ADD, ADHD and anger. Do these features result from distractions and excessive attention due to the presence of tics? Further, do these co-morbidities improve when tics decline spontaneously or in response to medication?

Many studies have supported an association between clinically referred individuals with TS and psychiatric symptoms and/or disorders, such as anxiety, ADHD and explosive outbursts or rage attacks. In understanding the etiology of non-tic symptoms in individuals with TS, it is important to distinguish normal emotion from symptom from disorder. Anxiety and anger, for example, are within the spectrum of normal emotional response which can occur in all individuals, but may be experienced at higher rates or more intense levels in individuals with TS. Anxiety and anger, especially at higher levels, may also occur as symptoms of a variety of psychiatric disorders, such as OCD, separation anxiety disorder, oppositional defiant disorder or a mood disorder. Symptoms of hyperactivity, reduced concentration, distractibility and/ or impulsivity, which impact academic, interpersonal or occupational functioning, are the core features of ADHD, and may often co-occur with anxiety, anger and poor frustration tolerance.

Although the presence of tics in an individual with TS may result in temporarily reduced concentration, or emotional reactions of anxiety or anger, tics do not necessarily cause these features, since there are alternative explanations for their etiology. It is often the case that anxiety, anger and reduced concentration resulting directly from tics can be attenuated with effective treatment of the tics themselves. However, if the anxiety, anger or reduced concentration are symptoms of an anxiety or mood disorder or ADHD, then tic treatment alone is not usually enough to reduce these symptoms. Interestingly but not surprisingly, treatment of some co-morbid symptoms or disorders, such as anxiety, may also secondarily reduce the tics. More research is needed to disentangle many of these symptoms and features.

(Barbara J. Coffey, M.D.; Inside TSA; Fall 2011)

12. I have heard of some people referring to mental tics. Do these exist? If so what are they?

Tourette syndrome is defined by the presence of tics (which are repetitive behaviors), not be repetitive thoughts. There are lots of ways to describe how and why tic behaviors are repetitive. You may hear the words "stereotyped," "choreographed," patterned," "repertoires," "repeated," and other terms to describe the behaviors. These words characterize an important quality of tics—they are performed over and over again in identical (or nearly identical) ways in a person with TS, although no two people with TS are affected exactly in the same way as each other. Yet while TS is defined by the behavior, the behaviors are almost always caused by feelings (and perhaps also by thoughts), and these, too, are repetitive.

Most people who are formally diagnosed with TS also have related brain developmental and behavioral features that are not tics. Many of these related features are also performed in a repetitive way, just as the tics are. And some of these repetitive behaviors, like tics, are caused by repetitive thoughts.

One such feature can be seen in obsessions and compulsions. Many, and perhaps most, people diagnosed with TS also have some degree of obsessions (which are repetitive thoughts or mental images) and compulsions (which are repetitive behaviors different from tics). For some people with TS, these obsessive-compulsive features may disrupt well-being and activities of daily living or occur frequently enough that a formal diagnosis of OCD is also identified.

Both tics and compulsions are behaviors that, for most people who have either or both diagnoses, are performed repetitively in patterns. And neither tics nor compulsions are truly "involuntary," although tics are usually described as involuntary movements. Rather, the person with TS and/or the person with OCD usually perform tics and/or compulsions on purpose because of a related feeling, thought, or mental picture that makes it uncomfortable and intolerable not to perform the behavior. The discomfort is hard to ignore, and performing the action in a very precise, patterned way helps get rid of the discomfort, at least for a time. The length of time the relief lasts may be very brief (as brief as a split second) or may be very prolonged (lasting minutes or even hours).

But the feeling or thought or mental image does return, and it feels or seems pretty much the same way each time it occurs. And the most effective, and often the only way to relieve this feeling or thought or unpleasant mental picture is by performing the tic or the compulsion in nearly exactly the same way, time and again. Despite this similarity in repetitive behavior between TS and OCD, there are important differences between the repetitive experiences (sometimes thoughts, sometimes not thoughts) that accompany TS and OCD, so let's consider these differences more fully.

First, let's consider TICS. If the unpleasant repetitive feeling occurs in the muscles that surround the eye, then an eye-blink tic may be the only patterned behavior that gives the person some relief. An example of this feeling that most people can understand is the sensation one feels when trying not to blink, such as when playing "the staring game." You will feel your eyelids grow heavy, your eyes may water up, and you will feel pressure or tickling around your eyes. You can keep yourself from blinking for a minute or so, but eventually the sensation is unbearable and you will give in. Blink. Relief at last! But in tics, these feelings build even when not trying to keep oneself from blinking, and similar feelings may also occur elsewhere in the body. If, for example the unpleasant feeling occurs together in the shoulders, waist and throat all at once, then a combination of shoulder shrugging an bending forward at the waist and grunting from the back of the throat may be the precise needed behavior repertoire (i.e., combination or sequence of behaviors) that allows a moment of relief.

Now, let's consider COMPULSIONS as different, but related, experiences. If an unpleasant repetitive thought (i.e., obsession) occurs, such as the idea that one's own hands are not clean, then washing one's hands may be the only patterned behavior that gives the person some relief. The person washed until the feeling is relieved, then stops washing, until he thought or feelings returns and builds up again.

While it often seems apparent that a repetitive behavior is either a tic or a compulsion, the distinctions can and do blur, and sometimes the repetitive feelings and the repetitive thoughts that cause the repetitive behaviors co-occur. For instance, a repeated sensation of sticky syrup between the fingers may accompany the repetitive idea of the hands being unclean. The combination of the sensation plus the idea can be intolerable.

Because both tics and compulsions share the feature of having an unpleasant repetitive experience (i.e., a feeling in tics, and an obsession in OCD) followed by a repetitive behavior to reduce the unpleasant experience (i.e., a tic or a compulsion), even very experienced professionals may not know for certain which is which. Some may somewhat jokingly use the name "compultic" in such cases.

Does using the correct name matter? It may. Where tics are caused by unpleasant sensations, whereas compulsions are caused by unpleasant ideas, what is going on in the brain may be quite different between the two. Unlike tics, obsessions and compulsions share a lot in common with anxiety. Anxiety is experienced as worry or unpleasant doubt or nervousness, and while anxiety may cause tics to become more frequent or severe, the anxiety is not the experience of the feelings behind the tics. Anxiety, however, is largely the experience in obsessions.

Some compulsions appear "tic-like" (e.g., tapping one's fingers hard onto a surface until relieved of the burden of the unpleasant feeling in one's fingertips that compel the person to tap) and other compulsions appear "anxiety-like" (e.g., tapping one's fingertips precisely 17 times because the repetitive thought that one must tap exactly 17 times is not relieved until 17 taps have been completed). Treatments available to reduce tics are generally poorly effective in reducing obsessions and compulsions. Treatments that are available to reduce obsessions and compulsions, however, may also be reasonably effective in reducing tics in people who have both tics and anxiety.

(Samuel H. Zinner, M.D; Inside TSA; Fall 2010)

13. Does everyone with TS utter obscene language (coprolalia)?

Definitely not! The fact is that less than one person in ten ever experiences Coprolalia. Too often, for its sensational effect, the media portray people with TS as shouting obscenities and ethnic slurs.

Coprolalia is a complex vocal tic that occurs when a person involuntarily repeats curse words, makes reference to male or female body parts, and utters racial epithets or other socially inappropriate vocalizations.

These unfortunate outbursts are by no means an indication of a person's personal beliefs. In the past, coprolalia was considered to be the defining feature of TS. Today, we no longer believe that having this symptom is necessary in order to confirm a TS diagnosis. Indeed, experienced clinicians agree that coprolalia is relatively uncommon among people with TS. This change in viewpoint is a reflection of the gradual broadening of the very definition of TS. Although it is not uniformly the case, coprolalia does tend to occur in those with the more severe forms of TS symptoms.

The cause of coprolalia is not known. However, the tics of TS—even simple tics—may challenge the boundary between what is voluntary and what is involuntary. This challenge is even greater when we try to understand more complex tics such as coprolalia.

Many, in fact most individuals with TS describe a feeling or an urge prior to performing some or all of their tics. Some will go even further and report that the feeling or urge actually drives the need to tic. They tell us that "If I didn't have the urge, I wouldn't have the tics." Generally, tics appear to be caused by a failure to inhibit signals in motor pathways in the brain. These pathways can be thought of as circuits or loops involving both sensory inputs (perhaps the source of premonitory urges) and motor outputs (movements). The actual physical location of the tic (e.g., facial movement, head jerk, shoulder shrug, throat clearing) may reflect the specific brain circuit where this failure of inhibition occurs. In other words, the reason why some people have facial tics and others have head jerks or throat clearing may have to do with the specific brain circuit that is not properly regulated. Putting this all together, we can imagine a person with TS feeling tension in the neck, followed very soon thereafter with a head jerking tic. There may be momentary relief from the tension—only to have it return again, and then the cycle repeats. Despite the very brief warning or feeling prior to the tic, we regard the movement as being involuntary because the person cannot stop the tic from occurring. In other words, an awareness that the tic is about to be expressed does not mean that the person can stop it from happening.

This model works pretty well for understanding simple motor and vocal tics. When it comes to complicated ones such as combination tics (e.g., a head jerk followed by an arm jerk and a grunting sound) or coprolalia, it gets—well—complicated. Once again, often people report a feeling or warning prior to executing a verbal outburst. Given that coprolalia involves motor output (muscles used in speech) and the production of a word that has meaning and that is socially inappropriate—it seems likely that more than one brain pathway or circuit is involved.

(Lawrence Scahill, Ph.D.; Inside TSA; Spring 2008)

14. Is there a connection between TS, rage and anger? How can parents and physicians manage these behaviors?

Anger is one of the basic human emotions; people report that they are angry about once or twice per week, and that on average, their anger lasts about thirty minutes. Anger varies in intensity from mild annoyance to rage and fury. People express this emotion in different ways—some ways are adaptive, such as finding a solution to the problem that caused anger, and other ways are far less acceptable socially such as yelling or hitting another person. Throughout the course of our development and socialization, we all learn how to control excessive experiences and maladaptive expressions of anger. However, frequent and very intense anger, particularly when it is accompanied by yelling, pushing or throwing things, creates a problem not only for those who experience it, but also for those who are the targets of these outbursts.

Children, adolescents, and adults with TS, particularly those who seek clinical attention, often report levels of anger that are higher than in the general population. For example, in a survey of 3,500 adults with TS, anger was noted as a problem by 37 percent of the participants. Anger, aggression and obstinacy are reported by the parents of 60 percent of children with TS who seek clinical services. Due to their intensity and unpredictability in response to minimal provocation, anger outbursts in TS have been described as rage attacks or rage storms. The explosive and out-of-character nature of anger outbursts in TS resembles the characteristics of aggression noted in intermittent explosive disorder as well as with what has been described as anger attacks in depression.

Whether excessive anger is actually a part of having TS, or related to co-occurring conditions, or due to the burden of coping with a chronic illness, is not clear. Moreover, the relationship between tic severity and anger is difficult to study due to the waxing and waning nature of tics. That said, frequent and intensive anger outbursts may prove to be a marker of more severe forms of TS. The best-documented research finding to date indicates that having ADHD in addition to TS may be contributing to disruptive behavior and anger outbursts in children with TS. Also, it may be that brain mechanisms that underlie impulse control and emotion regulation are somehow affected in TS, but these areas of research are still awaiting investigation.

There are a number of strategies parents can use to help their children control anger. One of the best-known behavioral treatments for child disruptive behavior, including anger and aggression, is called "Parent Training." This method teaches parents how to reduce the frequency and intensity of their child's outbursts. The core skills include providing positive reinforcement for appropriate behavior, communicating directions effectively, and being consistent with consequences for disruptive behaviors.

Different resources that parents and mental health professionals can use to learn about this treatment include Alan Kazdin's "Parent

Management Training" (Oxford 2005) or Russell Barkley's "Defiant Children" (Guilford 1997). Parent training programs may consist of 8 to 12 weekly, one-hour sessions. About 60 percent of parents report a significant reduction in their child's disruptive behavior.

"Anger Control Training" is another type of cognitive behavioral therapy that we have evaluated in adolescents with TS who exhibit excessive anger. This involves ten weekly sessions that include education about emotion regulation, problem solving, and role-playing of appropriate behaviors that can be used in frustrating situations. For example, as part of the problem solving training, children have to identify and evaluate the consequences of various actions for themselves and for the others involved in hypothetical conflicts. After that, a child can be asked to recall a time when he or she was frustrated, and then is asked to problem solve and role play behaviors that would have de-escalated the problem. At the end of each session, children are assigned homework to practice particular "anger coping" skills and to write about their positive anger management experiences. These reports are then discussed at the next session.

Both Parent Training and Anger Control Training are examples of psychosocial interventions that have been studied and shown to be effective in children without tics. We have recently completed two studies of these interventions in children and adolescents with TS complicated by explosive and disruptive behavior. One study evaluated the effects of Parent Training for 6 to 11-year-old children, and the second one evaluated the effects of Anger Control Training for 12 to 16-year-old adolescents. We reasoned that difficulties in family interactions on the one hand, and problems with the child's emotion regulation skills on the other hand, may contribute to disruptive behavior seen with TS. This is no different than what has been observed among people who do not have TS. Although the samples were small, our results were encouraging and suggest that both Parent Training and Anger Control Training may help to reduce disruptive behavior in children and adolescents with tics. However, larger studies are needed to confirm these results.

There are several signals that indicate when anger outbursts may require clinical attention. These may include danger to self or others, property damage, high frequency, duration and intensity of episodes, as well as disruption in family life, school achievement, and peer relations.

The root causes of anger outbursts in TS are poorly understood. Therefore, when children and adolescents with TS are brought to clinical attention, anger outbursts may be mistakenly attributed to their having TS, and unfortunately, co-occurring conditions such as ADHD may be overlooked. Also, these outbursts may pose a dilemma for clinicians who must decide whether to focus treatment on the tics (the core characteristic of TS) or on disruptive behavior problems. Careful evaluation of disruptive behavior and associated psychopathology should be among the first steps when planning treatment for these youngsters.

Regarding the treatments we have studied in our Yale TS clinic and seeking a professional provider, there is a good chance that behaviorally trained mental health professionals with different specialties such as psychology, social work, nursing, and psychiatry may well have expertise in Parent Training and Anger Control Training. It is possible that your doctor may be able to make a referral. Alternatively, you may contact mental health providers on your medical insurance list, and inquire about their experience with behavioral treatments for disruptive behavior.

(Denis G. Sukodolsky, Ph.D.; Inside TSA; Spring 2007)

15. My 10-year-old son has TS. Lately, he has become very aggressive and is acting out of character. He used to be a well-behaved child. Now he has temper tantrums and acts out a lot. How can I determine whether or not my son's sudden temper tantrums are TS related or just ordinary temper tantrums that children sometimes have?

It can be difficult to distinguish between ordinary temper tantrums and aggression that is part of an actual disorder. Typically, frequency, severity and duration are less with temper tantrums or there may be a readily identifiable environmental cause such as pressure and stress at home, in school or with friends.

Pathologic aggression with or without tics may be associated with a mood disorder. These can include depression or mania. Depression in a child may be apparent from a sad or irritable mood or a persistent loss of interest or pleasure in the child's favorite activities. Other signs and symptoms include changes in appetite and weight, abnormal sleep patterns, fatigue, and diminished ability to think, as well as feelings of worthlessness or guilt or even suicidal preoccupation.

Classical mania in adults is characterized by euphoria, elation, grandiosity, and increased energy. However, in most children, mania is more commonly manifested by extreme irritability or explosive mood with associated poor social and academic functioning that is often devastating to the patient and family. In milder conditions, additional symptoms include un-modulated high energy such as a decreased sleep, over talkativeness, racing thoughts, or increased goal-directed activity (social, work, school, sexual) or an associated manifestation of markedly poor judgment such as thrill-seeking or reckless activities. Importantly, only a clinician can make definitive recommendations for your child.

(Thomas Spencer, M.D.; Inside TSA; Winter 2003)

16. Is there a relationship between Tourette Syndrome and other neurological disorders such as Autism and Asperger's?

A variety of abnormal movements including tics, stereotypies, and catatonia have been found in individuals with Autistic Spectrum Disorders. Compulsive symptoms and perseveration behaviors are also common in this population. It can be particularly difficult to distinguish among complex motor tics, mannerisms, and compulsions in some individuals with TS, but these distinctions can prove even more difficult to make in individuals with Autistic Spectrum Disorders. Studies that have looked at the co-occurrence of the two conditions have produced a broad range of results. For example, recent clinical studies suggest that the prevalence of TS in people with Autism Spectrum Disorders (ASD) appears greater than that in the general population. A 2007 study by Canitano and Vivanti examined a clinical sample of 105 children and adolescents with ASDs; 22% were found to have comorbid tics. Among these children with both ASD and tics, half met diagnostic criteria for TS and the other half had chronic motor tic disorders. In this particular study, an association between the level of mental retardation and tic severity was reported. A much smaller study by Ringman and Jankovic in 2000 evaluated 12 patients with ASD that were referred to a movement disorders clinic. (Clinic referrals are markedly different from those sampled from the general community.) They found that half met diagnostic criteria for TS. A larger community sample of 447 children studied by Baron-Cohen et al. in 1999 indicated that approximately 6.5% of children had combined ASD and TS.

It should be noted that tic symptoms are noted in a range of neurobehavioral conditions. The study of the phenomenology and physiology of symptoms that commonly co-occur in a variety of these neurodevelopmental disorders such as Asperger's Syndrome, Tourette syndrome and ADHD and others remains an area of active research.

(Cathy L. Budman, M.D.; Inside TSA; Summer 2008)

17. For some time I've wondered whether or not TS is similar to other movement disorders such as Parkinson's disease or Dystonia.

Movement disorders are neurological syndromes where there is either an excess of movement or paucity of movement. This can apply either to voluntary or automatic movement. The prototype disease entity for poverty or paucity of movement is Parkinson's disease. TS, on the other hand, is an example of a movement disorder, with excessive involuntary movements. Movement disorders are classified together because, for the most part, they arise from the same area in the brain, namely the Basal Ganglia. Moreover, malfunction of the same chemical substances (neurotransmitters) in the brain is associated with the different movement disorders. For example, malfunction in dopamine regulation is involved in both Parkinson's disease and Tourette, with Parkinson's disease being associated with low dopamine levels and TS associated, among other abnormalities, with hyper-function of dopamine. It should be noted that even though movement disorders do share a common basis in some ways, having one does not make a person vulnerable to having another. Therefore, even if individuals have TS, as they age they are not at a higher risk for Parkinson's disease.

(Katie Kompoliti, M.D.; Inside TSA, Spring 2009)

18. My brother has TS and now my son, who has just turned 6 six years old, has started to stutter when he speaks. Could this be a tic?

Indeed, it could be a tic symptom. In addition to the common vocal tics such as throat clearing, grunting, hooting, barking or even words or short phrases, some individuals with TS have speech irregularities.

These may include sudden changes in the pitch, volume, or tone of speech as well as what we call blocking in speech. In some cases, this blocking can resemble stuttering. In some cases, telling the difference between speech blocking, tics, and stuttering may be difficult. Past history may help. For example, a child who had a history of stuttering prior to the onset of tics would suggest a return of the stuttering. On the other hand, a child with no prior history of stuttering but who suddenly exhibits a speech dysfluency might suggest a speech blocking tic. Another potentially useful way to differentiate between stuttering and speech blocking tics is to ask about the presence of a premonitory urge prior to the speech problem. This split second urge or warning just prior to the blocking is more consistent with tic phenomenology than with stuttering. It should be noted, however, that the absence of a premonitory urge is not sufficient reason to rule out the possibility of a speech blocking tic. Referral to an experienced Speech Pathologist may help with a differential determination.

So what can be done? First, someone might reasonably ask: "if it is a tic—won't a TS medication stop the tic—proving that it was a tic all along?" With the possible exception of botulinum toxin injections, tic suppressing medications focused on a single tic symptom are often disappointing. When successful, tic suppressing medications do reduce tic severity generally. Individual tics may be decreased—but not eradicated. To make matters even more confusing, some of the same medications used for tics are used to treat stuttering. Two avenues might be worth pursuing: medication and behav¬ioral treatment. Careful discussion with the treating clinician about whether your child's tics warrant medication is appropri¬ate—bearing in mind that tic eradication is unlikely. Consultation with a speech pathologist may not only help with the differential diagnosis, it may also open up treatment options. Behavioral interventions have been developed for stuttering. These approaches may be especially useful if the consensus of your treating clinician, the consulting speech pathologist and you and your son is that the dysfluency is indeed due to stuttering.

(Lawrence Scahill, Ph.D.; Inside TSA; Summer 2007)

19. I have a son with TS who has told me that he feels a cramp or spasm in his stomach. I have heard some people say that this is a stomach tic. Do stomach tics exist or is this possibly something that is stemming from a different condition?

Tics can appear in many parts of the body, especially the upper part of the body. Abdominal muscles can be a site of motor tics. The stomach is a digestive organ within the abdominal cavity. Many people refer to the abdominal muscles as their stomach. Are you referring to this digestive organ or the abdominal muscles? Tics within the digestive organ—the stomach—would not be expected to be involved in TS.

(Stanley Fahn, M.D.; Inside TSA; Winter 2010)

20. My son does something which can be disturbing to many people he pulls people's hair. He then laughs about it. I have heard that kids with TS often feel remorseful when they do things like this but he doesn't seem to feel that way. Can this be a tic that he is masking with laughter?

First, does your son have motor or vocal tics? Does he have TS? If so, then pulling someone's hair could be part of his tic behavior. Even if he has TS, pulling someone's hair could be a behavior problem. If he doesn't have TS, and just pull's someone's hair, it is likely this is a behavioral problem and not a tic.

(Stanley Fahn, M.D.; Inside TSA; Winter 2010)

21. I have seen people who constantly blink their eyes and recently learned that eye blinking is a common tic. Is there a difference between rapid eye blinking, eye twitching and tics?

Eye blinking in a child is usually a tic. Eye blinking in an older adult is usually a condition known as blepharospasm, which is another motor disorder. Blepharospasm is listed in the category of the dystonias, and is a dystonia of the eyelids. Dystonia can appear in many parts of the body, and it is fairly common in the eyelids.

(Stanley Fahn, M.D.; Inside TSA; Winter 2010)

22. I know someone who says that he has something called a Myoclonic jerk but to me it looks like a tic; are these two the same?

Myoclonic jerks are another movement disorder, separate from tics. Myoclonic jerks are always simple movements, not complex ones. Tics can be either simple or complex. If tics are only simple, they resemble myoclonic jerks. A movement disorder neurologist should be able to distinguish between the two conditions.

(Stanley Fahn, M.D.; Inside TSA; Winter 2010)

23. How many people in the U.S. have TS?

Tourette syndrome was initially thought to be a very rare disorder. However, patients with this syndrome have been identified in every country and geographic area in which researchers have looked for them. Tourette syndrome affects all ethnic groups, although for reasons that remain unclear, the disorder seems to be approximately 50% less prevalent in African American and sub-Saharan black African populations than in other groups. Boys are 3-4 times more likely to develop Tourette syndrome than girls. The estimated prevalence (occurrence) of tics and Tourette syndrome in children varies widely and there is no clear rate for adults. Several epidemiological studies suggest that up to 24% of children develop tics at some time during their childhood. Several studies have reported 1-30 (0.1-3.0%) cases of Tourette syndrome per 1,000 children, although rates of 0.3-0.8% are thought to best reflect the occurrence of the disorder. The Centers for Disease Control and Prevention reported that three of every 1,000 (0.3%) school-age children (that is, aged 6-17 years) in the US have Tourette syndrome. Analyses of data from epidemiological studies suggest that the overall prevalence of this disorder in most countries could be as high as 1% of children.

(Kevin McNaught, Ph.D. and Jonathan Mink, M.D., Ph.D.; Nature Review Neurology; 2011)

24. How does a person get Tourette Syndrome?

Although Georges Gilles de la Tourette suggested an inherited nature for Tourette syndrome, the precise pattern of transmission and identification of the gent remain elusive. Strong support for a genetic disorder is provided by studies of twins that show an 86% concordance rate for Tourette syndrome or other chronic tic disorders in monozygotes compared with 20% in dizygotes. A proposed gender-influenced, autosomal-dominant role if inheritance with variable expressivity as Tourette syndrome, chronic tic disorder, or OCD has been more recently replaced by hypotheses of a single major locus in combination with a multifactorial background, i.e., either additional genes or environmental factors. To date, no specific locus has been identified in large multigenerational families. A recent study in sib-pairs with Tourette syndrome has shown suggestive, but not significant, lod scores for two regions, 4q and 8p. In the future, important results should be generated from linkage studies on additional sib-pairs and isolated populations, such as Afrikaner, French Canadian, Icelandic, and Ashkenazi Jewish populations. It seems likely, however, that several genes are involved with the transmission of this disorder.

A variety of environmental factors have been proposed but not proven to be etiologic or modifying agents, including low birth weight, conditions influencing intrauterine growth, exposure to medications or illicit drugs, hyperthermia, and infections (most notable, streptococcal). The possibility that tics can occur as a post-infectious autoimmune disorder associated with a streptococcal infection (PANDAS—Pediatric Autoimmune Neuropsychiatric Disorders Associated with Streptococcus) is derived from several sources: reports of tics as a sequel to Sydenham chorea, evidence suggesting that Sydenham chorea may be mediated by streptococcal antibodies that cross-react with the brain, observation of a temporal relationship between streptococcal infection and the abrupt onset and exacerbation of OCD and tics, serologic testing showing elevation of antistreptolysin O in some abrupt onset tic patients, presence of antineuronal antibodies in children with movement disorders, and case reports of improvement of tics and OCD after plasma exchange or the use of intravenous immunoglobulin. Nevertheless, the existence of this entity is controversial, and additional studies are in progress to clarify the validity of PANDAS.

(Harvey Singer, M.D.; 10 Most Commonly Asked Questions About TS; The Neurologist; Vol. 6, No. 5; September 2000)

25. My child has just been diagnosed with TS at age 10. Neither my husband nor I have any family members with TS. We were told that TS is a hereditary disorder. How can that be if we do not have any relatives with this condition in our family?

Your question is a very common one because so many descriptions of TS do mention the role of genetics as a significant risk factor in causing this disorder. While the role played by genetics is not disputed and even though the evidence is growing that point to specific genetic risks, nevertheless, it is less well appreciated that the majority of close relatives of people with TS do not have medical histories of having TS symptoms themselves. This holds true for other closely associated disorders such as OCD.

So, how can we explain this absence of affected relatives when the disorder is known to be genetic? We believe that in order for youngsters to develop 'classic' and diagnosable TS, they must possess multiple risk factors which, when added together, contribute sufficient risk for developing TS. Following up on this idea, it makes sense that many individuals may carry some of these risk factors, but are free of the symptoms of the disorder. In other words, it is only when multiple risk genes plus other factors come together (perhaps being contributed from both sides of the family) that sufficient risk to develop the disorder occurs.

Moreover, there are some professionals who believe that for TS to develop, a genetic risk must be "activated" by a life experience (environmental cause) of some kind—e.g. in utero conditions, birth injury, or possibly certain infections. These theories have been studied to some extent, but we do not have definitive data as yet. So, we can understand that the path to developing TS can be quite complex and therefore not readily understood by just looking at the manifestation of TS symptoms among our family relatives.

(James T. McCracken, M.D.; Inside TSA, Fall 2008)

26. I am the father of identical twin boys with Tourette Syndrome. I met a man in his sixties who doesn't have TS, but his identical twin brother does. What do you know about the prognosis of TS in cases where there are twins?

Most of what we know about TS in twins comes from a few, relatively small studies of TS and tic disorders carried out with siblings. These studies indicate that about 50-70% of identical twin pairs (with the same genetic endowment) will both have TS. In the other 30-50% of identical twin pairs, only one of the twins will express the disorder. Concordance rates (meaning cases where both twins have the same syndrome or symptom) are higher for tic disorders in general. In 70-95% of identical twins where one twin has some type of tic disorder (including TS), the other twin will also have a tic disorder. Also, we've learned that in families where both twins have TS or another chronic tic disorder, one twin's symptoms may be more severe than the other. It is thought that these differences in severity may be associated with a variety of environmental factors. For example, in one study, the identical twins who had more severe symptoms also had lower birth weights than their co-twins with milder symptoms.

In other words, twin studies suggest that although TS is an inherited condition, there is a great deal of variability in the expression of TS, and this variability is likely due, at least in part, to environmental factors. As far as we know, the prognosis of TS, that is, the way the disorder develops, progresses, or improves over time, is no different in twins than in other people.

(Carol Mathews, M.D.; Inside TSA; Winter 2009)

27. My Husband and I are debating whether or not to have a child. He has TS and doesn't want to put a child through what he suffered growing up. What is the likelihood that our child will have TS?

TS is a genetic disorder that can be passed from one generation to the next. Since your husband has TS there is approximately a 50% chance that your child would inherit the genetic vulnerability for TS. However, not all children with this genetic vulnerability actually develop tics or other symptoms.

The exact odds are dependent on other factors including the gender of the child (males are more likely to develop symptoms). In addition, there is no way to predict the severity of your child's symptoms on the basis of your husband's tics.

I suggest that you consult with a reputable genetic counselor. Such counseling will provide you with precise information, and help you deal with the complex emotions associated with this important decision.

(John Piacentini, Ph.D.; Inside TSA; Winter 1998)

28. I am concerned that taking the flu vaccine will cause me to develop tics

It would be a shame if you yourself came down with a bad case of the flu, and then unwittingly transmitted it to someone who might actually die from this viral infection. Concerns about vaccines generally require balancing the risks of this preventative medical intervention versus the risks of contracting a disease. Sometimes the risks for individuals can differ depending on whether a person has a particular chronic medical condition. Fortunately, for healthy people with TS, the risks of unwanted effects are no greater than average. That is why we advise families that having TS does not put someone at greater risk when making decisions about whether or not to be vaccinated.

Here are two bottom lines for consideration: Individuals—if you are not vaccinated, you are more likely to get sick. Populations—if our citizens choose not to vaccinate, millions more people will become sick and unfortunately that includes some who will die.

Above all it is important to work with a well-informed primary care physician and also to consult a reliable source of information, such as the U.S. Centers for Disease Control website.

(Donald L. Gilbert, M.D.; Inside TSA; Spring 2010)

29. Is there a cure for TS?

There is no cure for TS yet, but treatments to reduce tic severity and the symptoms of other related conditions can be very effective.

30. People with TS take a variety of medication that were originally developed to treat other conditions, e.g. anti hypertensives, typical and atypical neuroleptics, etc. Why are these drugs effective for some people, some of the time and not others?

The late Arthur Shapiro M.D., one of the first physicians of the modern era to study TS, said that "every medication has made tics better and every medication has made tics worse." It is important to understand this basic truth. Many medications used for TS were initially observed to be successful only later to be studied more rigorously and found to be less effective than originally thought.

Two groups of medications have been consistently found to be successful in reducing tic symptoms. The first group is the neuroleptics, such as haloperidol or pimozide. These medications were tried in TS in part because of clinical "hunches" that they might reduce tics. The neuroleptics are involved in dopamine metabolism and dopamine is central to movement control. Similarly, the use of alpha adrenergic agonists, such as clonidine, was based on its effect on the overall central nervous system arousal level and brain functioning. There were also preliminary data suggesting that it might be useful in treating ADHD and might not necessarily result in changes in tic severity. Guanfacine, which is similar to clonidine, was tried in TS in part because it appeared to address inattention better than clonidine, and because it could be given two times a day as opposed to three to four times per day for clonidine.

No one treatment is effective for everyone. Individual response is likely determined by many factors—only one of which is specific neurochemical activity. Much more research needs to be done to identify both clinical characteristics associated with clinical response, but also genetic and neurological factors that are associated with tic severity as well as an individual's response to medication.

(John Walkup, M.D.; Inside TSA; Fall 2002)

31. Can stimulant medications used in the treatment of ADHD either cause Tourette Syndrome or worsen TS symptoms?

The misconception that stimulant medications cause Tourette syndrome arose because typically, the symptoms of inattention and hyperactivity often begin about a year before the onset of tics. Therefore, frequently stimulant treatment is prescribed some months before the onset of tics. In the past, this sequence of events created the mistaken impression that there is a causal connection between taking stimulants and the onset of tics. Often careful medical history reveals that mild tics were actually present before treatment with stimulants was begun. In addition, studies of identical twins where only one twin was exposed to stimulants have shown that the second twin, who was not treated with stimulants, developed tics. In summary, the evidence shows that stimulants do not cause tics.

How do stimulants impact tic severity? Completed a couple of years ago a large study has found that stimulant treatment did not increase symptoms and that in fact in some individuals the tics in fact decreased after the stimulant treatment was begun. Although stimulants may worsen TS symptoms in some individuals, for a majority of TS patients they do not cause significant worsening of tics, the exacerbation is short lived, and therefore they can be taken safely and with good effect for those with ADHD symptoms.

(Paul Sandor, M.D.; Inside TSA; Winter 2006)

32. My daughter has TS and wants to get pregnant. Should she stop taking her TS medication?

Most drugs used in the treatment of tics are labeled by the FDA as pregnancy category C, that is, "animal studies show adverse fetal effect(s) but no controlled human study is available to assess this risk." The recommendation in these cases is "to weigh the possible (mostly unknown) fetal risk vs. maternal benefit." In other words, if the tics are mild, it is best to plan the pregnancy in such a way that the mother can be weaned off all medications prior to conception. After all, unlike epilepsy and diabetes, tics are generally not life threatening. However, if the tics are so bad that removing anti-tic medication will likely exacerbate them, thus making the experience of pregnancy more challenging, an individual decision has to be made with an obstetrician's and neurologist's help, and in some cases, a pediatrician with special training in assessing fetal risks. The question they will need to address: Is the risk to the pregnancy and the fetus that may result from increased tics likely to be higher than those that may result from taking these drugs? Again, this is always a case-by-case decision, particularly in light of the lack of specific guidelines for TS.

(Jorge L. Juncos, M.D.; Inside TSA, Fall 2005)

33. I am an adult, who was taking narcoleptic drugs for several years. After sometime I developed tics as a side effect. My doctor has diagnosed me with "Adult onset Tardive Tourettism" and I am confused because I have never had tics prior to taking these medications and I have read that TS is diagnosed before the age of 18. If it is not Tourette Syndrome then why do they call it Tourettism?

First, I suspect you are referring to "neuroleptic" drugs and not "narcoleptic" ones. Neuroleptic drugs can cause a number of neurologic side effects, including a condition known as "tardive dyskinesia," which is persistent abnormal movements that might disappear over time. Tardive dyskinesia can manifest in a variety of abnormal movements, including as tics, where it is called "tardive tics." Because tardive tics resemble the tics of Tourette syndrome, some doctors have called it "tardive tourettism."

(Stanley Fahn, M.D.; Inside TSA; Winter 2010)

34. What is CBIT and is it different from Habit Reversal Therapy (HRT) and Cognitive Behavioral Therapy (CBT)?

CBIT (Comprehensive Behavioral Intervention for Tics) is based on HRT—a behavioral treatment that has been studied and in use for many, many years. However, CBIT includes a number of methods that are not part of HRT but rather are specific to TS. For instance CBIT focuses primarily on increasing an awareness of tics and teaching individuals how to perform a competing behavior just when they sense the tic symptoms are about to occur.

Also, those who undergo this training are encouraged to become aware of and avoid tic-worsening triggers such as certain places, specific activities or even other people who might cause them stress. Once these triggers are recognized and avoided individuals can experience a decrease in symptoms. Participants in the CBIT program (both those with TS and their families) are also exposed to a great deal of education about tic disorders.

(Douglas W. Woods, Ph.D.; Inside TSA; Summer 2008)

35. Can TS symptoms be controlled by willpower?

The tics of TS are usually considered involuntary. However, that does not mean that the patient has absolutely no control over their tics. Indeed, even untreated patients are sometimes able to suppress their tics for various periods of time. Recent research disproved the old belief in a "rebound effect." In other words, we have learned that when a previously suppressed tic is finally allowed to come out, it is not stronger or longer lasting than usual.

Behavioral therapy for TS teaches patients various strategies to gain control over their tics. Patients are taught how to increase their awareness of tics, learn how to cope with factors that make their tics worse, and how to engage in substitute behaviors instead of expressing unwanted tics. They also learn relaxation exercises and engage in relapse prevention training to ensure that they can maintain their gains after therapy has ended.

The goal of this treatment is not to cure TS, but to teach the patients powerful tic management skills. Very encouraging is the fact that behavior therapy has now been evaluated in at least four controlled studies and all had positive results.

(Sabine Wilhelm, Ph.D.; Inside TSA, Winter 2008)

36. Is brain surgery used to treat Tourette Syndrome?

The answers are, "Yes" and "No":

Yes—experimental brain surgery has been done on a few very unusual cases of TS with extremely severe symptoms that cannot be reduced by medications. The surgery, called deep brain stimulation (DBS), involves placement of electrodes into areas of the brain believed to be important for movement control. A small number of adult TS cases have been described on television shows, with the misleading claim that DBS is a `cure.' A somewhat larger, but still overall small number of cases have been reported in the peer reviewed medical literature.

No—In the United States, DBS surgery is approved, by FDA for three conditions: Essential Tremor, Parkinson's Disease and Dystonia. It is currently being investigated for some other neurological and psychiatric conditions, however it is not approved for TS, and there are currently no large scale studies to determine whether DBS surgery is safe and effective for TS. In the vast majority of TS cases, consideration of trying brain surgery and implantation of electrical devices would not be appropriate.

(Donald L. Gilbert, M.D.; Inside TSA, Winter 2008)

37. At a recent TSA Chapter meeting, I heard people say that TS symptoms could be reduced by undergoing Botox injections. Is this true?

Botulinum toxin (Botox) is a very potent neurotoxin that in essence weakens/paralyzes muscles. The onset of the action is gradual, and it can last up to 3 to 6 months. Botox injections have been used for medical purposes since the early 1980s. The first use was in Strabismus, an ophthalmological disorder. Since the late 1980s Botox injections have been used for movement disorders like Dystonia and other medical conditions like spasticity, drooling, excessive sweating, bladder control and gastrointestinal problems. For some of these disorders, like cervical dystonia, Botox injections are FDA approved first line treatments. Therefore, neurologists have significant experience using Botox for medical purposes.

These injections have also been used in the treatment of tics. There is substantial anecdotal experience, a few uncontrolled studies and at least one well-designed, placebo-controlled study that concluded that Botox can be a useful tool in treating both motor and vocal tics.

However, Botox is a treatment that can only be used to target a specific area of the body. For example, if the patient has a single blinking tic, this could be a very beneficial treatment. Other areas that can be easily approached are shoulder and neck tics.

Botulinum toxin cannot be used to address the whole repertoire of an individual's tics, because of technical and dose limitations. In treating refractory vocal tics, vocal cord injections have been used with variable success. When treating tics with Botox injections, it has been noted that there is also a decrease in the urge that precedes the tics. Side effects are a result of weakening certain muscle groups and in the case of vocal cord injections include low volume voice (hypophonia), which frequently occurs in the first few weeks of treatment.

Administering Botox injections requires special expertise that is available only at specialized centers. Therefore, it is not always readily accessible to everyone. Finally, it is an expensive treatment and since the FDA has not approved this treatment for reducing tics, health insurance varies greatly among providers.

(Katie Kompoliti, M.D.; Inside TSA, Spring 2009)

38. My son is 8 yrs. old and was recently diagnosed with TS. We don't really want to put him on medication right now and are looking for other options. I am finding a lot of information on the internet and from other sources about nutritional therapy for TS symptoms. I have also heard about food and environmental allergies and how they can affect the brain. Are these useful avenues to pursue?

There is growing and very influential interest in "integrative healthcare" for childhood neurodevelopmental and behavioral conditions and general health. Often, integrative healthcare refers to "alternative and complementary" systems that use uncustomary or scientifically unproven approaches. Actually, quite a few proven and customary approaches started out as "alternative" but over time gained acceptance, often through research evidence.

Recent attention has focused on autism spectrum disorders and ADHD. However, there is appreciable interest in TS as well. TSA continues to respond to this interest by encouraging researchers to conduct good-quality scientific studies to help to answer questions about nutrition, environmental allergies and other integrative healthcare issues. These studies will eventually enable doctors and families to make informed decisions about healthcare practices. In the meantime, it is important to consider any information available regarding safety and efficacy of any healthcare approach in treating (or not treating) TS and related conditions.

The Internet provides a ready source of both information and misinformation about healthcare. At this time, there are neither restrictive and/or supplemental dietary interventions, nor environmental and/or food allergens that have been proven to have an impact on TS symptoms. Resources are available to help educate clinicians, researchers and consumers about integrative healthcare and TS. Contact TSA or its web site www.tsa-usa.org for an informational brochure, "Complementary and Alternative Medicine for Tourette Syndrome." Extensive information about integrative healthcare is also available through the National Center for Complementary and Alternative Medicine at http://nccam.nih.gov.

(Samuel H. Zinner, M.D.; Inside TSA; Spring 2008)

39. My nephew seems to be drinking alcohol excessively and smoking marijuana. He says he won't stop because he is "self-medicating." What is the best thing to say to him?

There is no scientific evidence that alcohol can be used to reduce tics. However, it is possible that drinking alcohol may lessen tics indirectly, through decreasing anxiety.

Case reports and at least one controlled study provide evidence that marijuana (Cannabis sativa) and delta-9-tetrahydrocannabinol, the major psychoactive ingredient of marijuana, can be effective in the treatment of tics and behavioral problems in TS. The effects of delta-9—tetrahydrocannabinol on cognitive function and its abuse potential overshadow any possible benefit for controlling symptoms.

In conclusion, both alcohol and marijuana are unproven treatments for TS. Furthermore, these substances create more problems than they solve. Beyond their addictive nature, their chronic use can create medical and neurological problems, which will be much more difficult to address than tics.

(Katie Kompoliti, M.D.; Inside TSA; Spring 2009)

40. I have heard that hypnosis has been helpful for some people with TS. To me it seems very confusing and I am extremely skeptical. Can someone explain to me if and how hypnosis can be at all useful for a person with TS?

Hypnosis is not sleep nor is it an unusual state of consciousness. It can be viewed as a state of hyper-focused attention with decreased peripheral awareness. In hypnosis, one can assert greater control over and influence aspects of experience normally considered beyond conscious control. For example, hypnosis to manage pain without drugs is an application with strong empirical support, highlighting one's ability to communicate with and deliberately control part of one's body. Hypnosis brings about a state of mind where a person's normal critical or skeptical nature is bypassed, thus allowing for acceptance of suggestions. This state of heightened receptivity for suggestions (induction) is developed with the cooperation of the individual. The suggestions can be delivered by a professional (hypnotist) or the individual can be taught to self-administer them (self-hypnosis). The induction is followed by the therapeutic intervention which consists of providing positive suggestions.

When addressing tics, participants in hypnotherapy are usually taught to discriminate their tics from other movements. Simultaneously, self-hypnosis training is started, using relaxation techniques and visual imagery for deepening of the trance. Improvement is sought by instructing the subjects to bring the relaxed feelings back with them when the session is over. Although hypnosis can be a powerful tool, it has not been adequately studied in TS. A recent study reported positive effects of self-hypnosis training on 33 children and adolescents. More solid evidence is still required, since this study assessed efficacy based on self-report of improvement and did not assess long term effect of self-hypnosis.

(Samuel H. Zinner, M.D. and Katie Kompoliti, M.D.; Inside TSA; Summer 2011)

41. Many people with TS have reported that exercise and other physical activities have reduced their tics. Are there studies that support this and how does it work?

The benefits of aerobic exercise are increasingly apparent in medicine, emotional health and wellbeing, and preventive health. There are many anecdotal reports of tic reduction benefits (and even some of tic worsening) resulting from exercise, but there are no published scientific studies examining exercise and impact on tics to determine "if" it works, much less "how." There have been several research studies looking at exercise among people with other developmental and behavioral challenges, such as with reading disabilities or attention deficit disorders. Results about possible benefits are not clear. TSA's website provides a useful publication by Mitzi Waltz titled, "Exercise, Sports and Tourette Syndrome: Potential Benefits Abound."

As a precaution, this and any related information should not be taken as medical advice. Anyone considering beginning an exercise program should consult with a qualified professional. Also, consider combining play and exercise into the family or individual lifestyle.

Paul Devore, a TSA Board member with TS, discusses his own beneficial experiences with exercise and self-esteem, in a video available on the TSA website under the "For Adults with TS" section, "Paul Devore on Self Esteem."

(Samuel H. Zinner, M.D. and Katie Kompoliti, M.D.; Inside TSA; Summer 2011)

42. I have come across some information about nutritional supplements and vitamins, a few even claiming to be given specifically for TS. It is difficult to know which are actually successful. Do you know if any natural supplements can have a negative impact on someone with TS or are they all safe? What can you tell me about these supplements and vitamins? Do any of them actually have a proven track record?

Many dietary supplements, herbs, vitamins, and minerals have been promoted to reduce motor and vocal tics as well as the associated conditions that might accompany Tourette syndrome including attention deficit hyperactivity disorder, obsessive compulsive disorder, oppositional defiant disorder, and anger outbursts.

Ningdong granule (ND), a traditional Chinese medicine compound, hyoscyamus and chamomilla, Pycnogenol and omega-3 fatty acids are some of the supplements that have been linked to treatment of tics or ADHD. Currently, none of them is proven to have a definite effect.

In 1994, Congress passed the Dietary Supplement Health and Education Act (DSHEA), which removed supplements from the same degree of scrutiny by the Food and Drug Administration (FDA) that is required for traditional medicines. The manufacturers do not have to prove to the FDA the safety and efficacy of supplements before they are marketed. Rather, it is up to the FDA to demonstrate that a dietary supplement or an herb is unsafe once it is already in the market. In a recent survey of 40 popular herbal dietary supplements, the Government Accountability Office found trace amounts of at least one potentially hazardous contaminant in 37 of the products tested. Some preparations have been found to contain heavy metals (lead, mercury, and arsenic), bacteria, environmental chemicals and drugs (caffeine, corticosteroids, benzodiazepines such as Valium and diuretics).

When deciding to start a supplement, one has to keep in mind that although many dietary supplements (and some prescription drugs) come from natural sources, "natural" does not always mean "safe." For example, the herbs comfrey and kava can cause serious harm to the liver. It is important therefore to look for reliable sources of information on dietary supplements. Further information is available at the U.S. Food and Drug Administration: http://www.fda.gov/Food/DietarySupplements/default.htm.

(Samuel H. Zinner, M.D. and Katie Kompoliti, M.D.; Inside TSA; Summer 2011)

43. I have read that the elimination of sugar and certain food dyes can help people with ADHD. Would it be good for people with TS to reduce or eliminate sugar intake and certain food dyes also? Are there diets that would be particularly advantageous to people with TS?

The saying "you are what you eat" has held the public's interest for decades, and certainly also holds quite a bit of truth. We as consumers have become more aware of where our food comes from, although there remains much mystery about the best food choices for our physical and mental health. Since half or more people clinically diagnosed with TS also are diagnosed with ADHD, we'll examine both conditions here.

Diet and TS
The possibility that food may affect behavior in people with ADHD came to public attention in 1975 when a pediatric allergist Dr. Benjamin Feingold suggested that some artificial food coloring (AFC) and flavoring,

some food preservatives and foods that contain salicylates (which are chemicals that occur naturally in some fruits and vegetables) seemed to adversely affect many children's behavior. Dr. Feingold suggested that the behavior in about half of children with ADHD improved when removing these ingredients from the child's diet. The "Feingold diet" as it came to be called did not include elimination of sugar, but the diet does include elimination of some artificial sweeteners.

Separate from the Feingold diet, another line of concern evolved about eating refined sugar and its possible association with ADHD behaviors, due to effects of a rapid rise in blood sugar level as the most popular explanation.

In the years since publication of Dr. Feingold's initial hypothesis, there have been several research studies that apply the Feingold diet or that eliminate refined sugar. Results from these studies help to clarify possible food-behavior associations.

Regarding the Feingold diet, most studies have not shown an association with ADHD. Some studies have shown a possible, but small, association, although these studies generally have had significant faults in the study design, and in March 2011, a panel of experts brought together by the FDA concluded that the available evidence does not support putting warning labels about risks for ADHD on foods that contain artificial coloring. Most published reviews of available studies agree that there may be a minority of particularly vulnerable children with ADHD who benefit from the Feingold diet, but that determining which children would benefit is difficult. One reviewer concludes that a trial elimination diet is appropriate for children with ADHD who haven't shown adequate response to usual treatment approaches or whose parents are interested to pursue the diet.

Sugar and TS

Reviews of research looking into refined sugars and possible impact on behavior in children with ADHD generally agree that there is no usual association. Two reviews (published in 1995 and in 1996), one that examined 12 studies and another that examined 23 studies, concluded that the evidence does not support an association between sugar and behavior in children with ADHD. However, one review recognizes that a small effect of sugar on behavior is theoretically possible and that it's not possible to rule out that the behavior of a special subset of children with ADHD could be sensitive to sugar. A 1994 study examined mothers and sons who felt their sons with ADHD were sensitive to sugar. All boys received a sugar substitute, but half of the mothers were deceived, being told that their sons had instead received sugar. All mothers watched their sons on videotape, and those who thought their sons had received sugar reported that their son's behavior was much more hyperactive after the "sugar" than did mothers who were correctly informed of their sons' receiving the sugar substitute, suggesting that a parent's expectation of a sugar-hyperactive association may bias her perception of her child's behavior.

Unlike ADHD, there is virtually no available research looking at diet impact on TS, so far with just a single published study examining this topic. The 2008 study was a survey completed in Germany offered to patients in a TS clinic and to members of TS self-help groups. The researchers found meaningful associations in the respondents' perceptions between worsening of tics and consumption of Coke, coffee, black tea, preserving agents, refined white sugar and sweeteners. The authors correctly caution that only double-blind placebo-controlled studies (in contrast to the survey design of their study) are suitable to make a reliable statement regarding efficacy of a treatment's impact on tics.

Nutritional Supplements and Diet
A U.S. survey design study in 2004 inquired about nutritional supplements (not diet) and tics. The survey was offered to members of the TSA NY and to a subscription list of a newsletter that explores complementary or alternative medicine treatments for neurological conditions. The researchers reported that nearly 90% of respondents use nutritional supplements to control tics, remarking that it was not possible to relate tic changes to any specific nutritional supplement. The authors correctly caution that the study is not intended to provide evidence of benefit, and they identify several important limitations.

Conclusion
What to make of these results? While most available research does not associate diet and behavior in ADHD, and while there is no reliable research information regarding diet and tics, a healthful diet is good advice for lots of reasons, whether relating to weight management,

diabetes or cancer risks among many others. Parents interested in considering dietary interventions for treating behaviors of ADHD and/or tics should receive accurate information from their health care providers and should consider consultation with a dietitian to ensure balanced good nutrition.

(Samuel H. Zinner, M.D. and Katie Kompoliti, M.D.; Inside TSA; Fall 2011)

44. Does Having TS limit job opportunities?

I have always taken the philosophical approach that my having TS is irrelevant and I think this is particularly true in the area of your career. People with TS are doctors, lawyers, actors, accountants . . . every profession. TS tics may limit an individual's choices but no more, and usually a lot less, than other qualities. Your talent, ambition, personality and discipline play a greater role in determining your potential success in any given field. Not your tics.

You may dream of taking center stage at the Metropolitan Opera House and sing along with Renee Fleming on your iPod, but unless you have the voice, musical ability and the drive and determination of a diva, you're unlikely to make it in opera. You might also have a mean jump shot, but if you stop growing at 5'9", your basketball career has limits. TS is a little like that one-octave range voice or your height, it's a part of you, but it doesn't define you.

Young people with TS should explore all their interests and talents and never let having TS inhibit their dreams. When it comes to career opportunities TS is just one, and I think a very small, factor in the equation.

(Paul A. Devore, M.D.; Inside TSA; Winter 2008)

45. How can I enlist my doctor to advocate on my behalf in other areas, e.g. at school, work, etc., and what type of documents should a physician provide for parents who need appropriate services and accommodations from their children's school?

Parents can work together with physicians and school personnel on the impact of having TS and its associated disorders on classroom performance. The physician should consider addressing a letter to the school principal or to the director of special education requesting a thorough psycho-educational evaluation. Ideally, that evaluation should include auditory processing, language processing, memory skills, executive function, and fine motor and visual motor impairment. A Functional Behavioral Assessment may also be advisable. It is recommended that the child should also be seen by an independent neuropsychologist who is certified as a school psychologist. The doctor is in a good position to provide documentation of tic severity, medications, and any thoughts about co-occurring ADHD and OCD symptoms. There is an entire section on TSA's website devoted to issues concerning education. It might be helpful to consult that valuable information.

(Cheston Berlin, M.D.; Inside TSA; Summer 2009)

46. In everything I've read about TS, we are told not to bring up TS tics and other behaviors with our children because drawing attention to symptoms can make them more self-conscious. I agree with that view. However, my daughter is unbelievably embarrassed by her symptoms, and won't talk about them at all. I would like to explain TS to her. Any advice as to how to go about it?

It is true that if you talk to your daughter about her tics, the problem of "suggestibility" might exacerbate her tics, but that doesn't mean you should avoid serious talks with her about TS.

Sit down with her in a place where she feels comfortable, just the two of you, so she won't be embarrassed. It is important that she understand she is not responsible for her tics. And that she is not "bad"—because they happen regardless of her desire to stop.

Don't force her to talk, but assure her that you will be there when she is ready for a discussion and that you won't expose her to the ridicule of other family members, friends, classmates, etc.

TSA has booklets and videos that may help her understand TS. Matthew and the Tics is a pamphlet for young children. The DVD "I Have Tourette's But Tourette's Doesn't Have Me" might help start a conversation with an older child or adolescent.

(Louise Kiessling, M.D.; Inside TSA; Summer 1998)

47. Please discuss the fear expressed by some parents that a diagnosis is tantamount to a label that will follow their child in school, work, and life in general.

The diagnosis of tics, or more specifically that of TS, may provoke considerable anxiety for both individuals with the symptoms as well as their loved ones. Often the only frame of reference many people may have about TS are the dramatic and disturbing tic symptoms in a depiction of someone with TS on television or in a movie. This is unfortunate because it causes unnecessary anxiety and distress because many people misunderstand the tics and sadly, they assume that a diagnosis of TS is tantamount to a life of social estrangement and disability. This is absolutely NOT true.

(Cathy L. Budman, M.D.; Inside TSA; Summer 2009)

48. Do tics occur during sleep?

Yes, both motor and phonic/vocal tics can occur during sleep, although tic severity is often less than during awaking periods.

(Kevin McNaught, Ph.D. and Jonathan Mink, M.D., Ph.D.; Nature Review Neurology; 2011)

49. What factors can worsen or improve the severity of tics?

Certain factors and events, such as stress, anxiety and fatigue, can increase the occurrence of tics, whereas others—such as tasks requiring concentration and motor skills, including musical and athletic performances and/or physical exercise—can reduce or even temporarily halt tics.

(Kevin McNaught, Ph.D. and Jonathan Mink, M.D., Ph.D.; Nature Review Neurology; 2011)

50. What does the Tourette Syndrome Association, Inc. do?

- Maintains an Internet web site (http://tsa-usa.org) to keep you informed and answer your questions
- Helps families in crisis through its Information and Referral Service
- Promotes public awareness and understanding of TS
- Develops and maintains state-by-state lists of doctors and allied professionals (e.g. psychologist, social workers, and counselors for referral purposes

- Maintains an active teacher education program and provides guidance to parents on effective lobbying strategies for IEP programs
- Organizes workshops and symposia for scientists, clinicians and others working in the field of TS. Increases the knowledge and sensitivity of health care professionals to TS through exhibits at conferences and dissemination of literature at national meetings.
- Represents the interests of members to the government on critical policy issues including orphan drugs, health insurance and employment
- Publishes a quarterly newsletter and produces brochures and video tapes that discuss in detail many of the topics of interest to families and friends. For a full list and description, please consult our web site at http://tsa-usa.org.

(John T. Walkup, M.D.; Questions and Answers about Tourette Syndrome; May 2006)

Some copies of this publication are disseminated through cooperative agreement award number 5U38DD000727-02 from the Centers For Disease Control & Prevention. The views expressed in written materials or publications do not necessarily reflect the official policies of the Department of Health and Human Services, nor does mention of trade names, commercial practices, or organizations imply endorsement by the U.S. Government or the Tourette Syndrome Association.

Please evaluate this resource at
http://www.surveymonkey.com/s/familyguideTS